THE 30-SECOND BODY

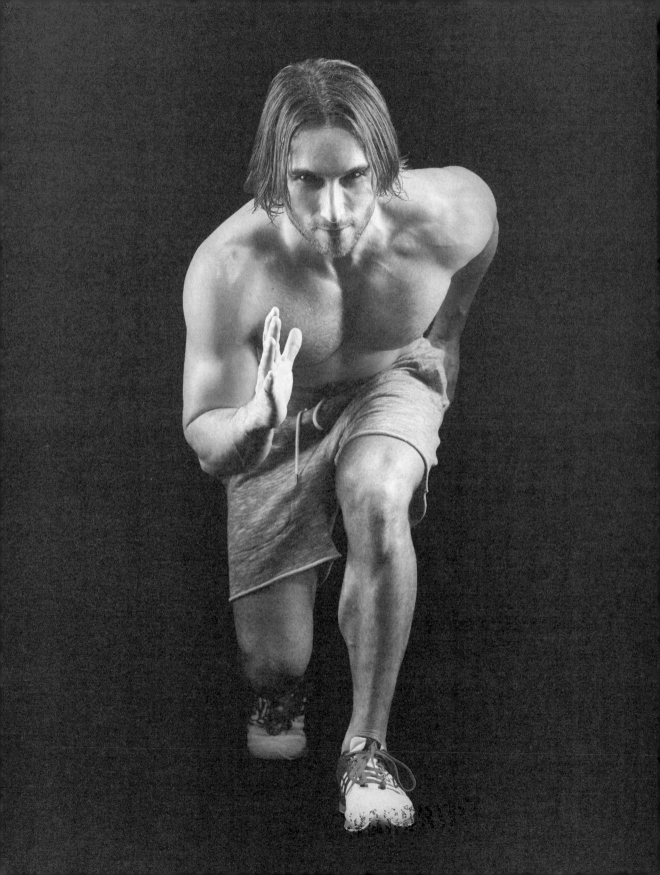

THE 30-SECOND BODY

EAT CLEAN. TRAIN DIRTY.
LIVE HARD.

ADAM ROSANTE

BALLANTINE BOOKS NEW YORK

A Zinc Ink Trade Paperback Original

Copyright © 2015 by Adam Rosante

Published in the United States by Zinc Ink, an imprint of Random House, a division of Random House LLC, a Penguin Random House Company New York.

BALLANTINE and the HOUSE colophon are registered trademarks of Random House LLC.

ZINC INK is a trademark of David Zinczenko.

ISBN 978-0-804-17920-1
eBook ISBN 978-0-804-17921-8

Printed in the United States of America on acid-free paper

www.ballantinebooks.com

9 8 7 6 5 4 3 2 1

Title-spread photograph: J. Ryan Roberts

To Kate. You are my *everything*. That I get to spend every day
with you makes me the luckiest man in the universe.

To Mom and Dad. All that I am, I owe to you. Thank you for
always believing in me and leading with your big-hearted,
sleeves-rolled-up example.

To Grandma. I miss you every day.

To Carissa. For teaching me the value of laughter, patience, and
love.

To Tom. Love you, buddy!

To little Leah. You can't read or walk yet, but girl, can you make
me smile. Seriously though, learn to read.

To Carl. For inspiring creativity and a sense of rebellion in me.

To my very large family, each and every one of you, for helping
raise me. I love you and can't express how fortunate I am that
there are too many of you to name here.

To Kevin. Thanks for *always* being there.

To all my friends. You know who you are and I'm speaking directly to each of you. You make my life the fun ride that it is.
XO.

And to you, dear reader. Thank you for choosing this book. You
are stronger than you think and capable of things you haven't
even begun to imagine.

CONTENTS

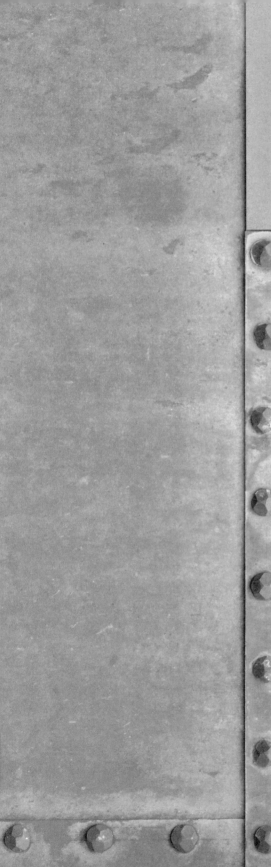

iNTRODUCTiON

RAISE YOUR HAND IF YOU'D RATHER SPEND your time laughing and enjoying a meal with your friends and family than suffering in a gym, starving yourself, or drinking some oddball potion to get in great shape.

Yup, my hand's up there, too.

You have in your possession the key to help you do just that. This book is going to help you unlock the body and life of your dreams without driving yourself crazy. Heck of a promise, I know; but it's one that I've been delivering on for more than ten years as a fitness trainer, nutrition coach, and wellness expert.

I'm known for my ability to make complicated and overwhelming information remarkably less so. That's why real people turn to me again and again to look and feel amazing. In 2012, I founded The People's Bootcamp, a pay-what-you-can fitness brand that is often referred to as the hardest workout in New York and that one magazine called "a populist antidote to the tyranny of $35 spin sessions." I also created WaveShape, a surf-inspired workout for some surfer friends, and then made it available for free online. It's used every day by thousands of people from Montana to Morocco.

You see, I like simplicity. No crap, no pomp, just the essentials: an effective plan and the tools to help you put it into play. Once you toss the rest, it's like a breath of fresh air.

Perhaps you've seen me on TV, sweating it out with your favorite morning show host; or you've read me doling out fitness tips in a magazine. Maybe you don't own a TV, haven't read an actual magazine in years, and think I'm just some crazy guy with a clever premise (that last part is definitely true!). Either way, I am 100 percent certain that by the time you get into these workouts, you'll be wondering how you could hate *and* love someone so much at the same time.

That's because I'm going to help you build a *30-Second Body*. Speaking of which, you're probably wondering just what that is.

Let me start with what it is not. The phrase *30-Second Body* does not mean that you only need to work out for thirty seconds a day to get in great shape. Sorry! It's not a magic trick or some infomercial gimmick, and it isn't a call to laziness.

But a *30-Second Body* is acquired quickly; a lot of people notice results after the first week. My style of working out is incredibly efficient and takes half as long as your average class at the gym. A *30-Second Body* is a physique that's built for speed, for show, for health, for life. It looks as good strutting down the runway as it does cruising down the produce aisle. Finish these workouts and you'll be sleek, crazy sexy, and know how to get in shape in less time than it takes to watch an episode of *Saved by the Bell*. Weird reference, I know. Keep reading. This book is filled with them!

A *30-Second Body* is long, lean, strong, agile, and fast. It torches calories while at rest—yes, *at rest*. It looks amazing; but best of all it functions like a well-oiled machine.

But don't worry: The program revealed in this book is not break-your-back, crazy-complicated, either. It's the ability to work out hard *and efficiently,* leaving a puddle of sweat on the floor as you proudly march forward into your day. It's a little gritty and a lot of fun.

So, how does it work?

I've chosen exercises that target your entire body, and stacked them into 30-second intervals to get you in amazing shape—*fast*! If you've heard of high-intensity interval training, this is it *at its finest*.

Yes, it's hard; but *yes,* you can do this. Over the next six weeks, you're going to unleash your best body. Are you ready?

Maybe you were once in awesome shape, but fell out of it for some reason or another. Perhaps you've always put fitness and wellness on the back burner, but have come to realize the importance of taking control of your body and getting it in killer shape. Or maybe you are already really fit, but looking to break through a plateau, lose those last ten pounds, or just try something new.

Whatever your life's journey, wherever you are right now, I'm going to help you get where you want to go. This book is going to give you the key to unlock your best body in record time, and keep it for life. It's also going to help you unleash your *mind.*

You'll prove to yourself that you're capable of far more than you ever imagined. That confidence stays with you. It goes beyond the confines of your sweat-soaked living room floor and into the world, helping you to live life to the fullest—to *live hard.* That's what I teach every day: strengthening both mind and body so that we can live "full out." The sweet physical results are just the cherries on top.

Is it going to be easy? No. Nothing worthwhile ever is. Is it going to be brutal? Depends on your definition of "brutal"—but know this: I designed this program with a wide variety of fitness levels in mind; so no matter how long it's been since you've worked out (and even if you *never have*), I guarantee that *you can do this*! I've seen people who haven't worked out in years step into one of my classes with fear in their eyes and leave with fire in their hearts.

The easy part is that this is a clear, simple-to-follow six-week workout plan that's going to melt fat, skyrocket your metabolism, and get you seriously toned up and strong. There's a free calendar (and a ton of other extras) at www.the30secondbody.com that you can print out and tack on your wall. There's also a tear-out version of that calendar in the back of this book. I'm giving you shockingly simple nutrition advice that'll kick fad diets to the curb. You'll eat awesome food five times a day and actually *enjoy* your life, without feeling like you're being restricted or made to go hungry. Finally, I'm going to show you how to rewire your mind so that you follow through and do the work needed to get in shape. Essentially, I've taken all the guesswork out of lifelong fitness and given you a road map.

So, what's the catch?

Well, the hard part is on you, I must admit, and it's *consistent effort*. If you want to grow an apple tree, I can give you a shovel and a sapling; but ultimately, you still have to dig the hole.

If it were as easy as just having a solid workout plan, everyone with access to the Internet would be trim and fit. So, why is it so hard for so many of us to get and stay in shape?

It's time to come to terms with a hard fact: We've been conditioned for failure since we were kids.

Whoa! Say what? It may feel like this book just took a hard left turn, but hang with me. Awareness is the first step toward change. I've found that most people aren't even aware of the choices they're making that sabotage their goals. I want you fit for life, not just sweating for a week or so and then abandoning me for some other program—which, inevitably, you'll abandon for another and another and another. Admit it. You're tired of that, and you're better than that. So let's be real.

For far too long we've been told we can have anything we want with zero effort. Get six-pack abs in fifteen minutes. Make $2 million a year in four hours a week. Look nineteen again with the latest, greatest miracle cream.

The companies making these pitches do their best to convince you that the only people who get results are the ones who are following the right plan, that is, *their* plan. To drive their point home, they often trot out a parade of "after" models who have gone from "drab to fab" to say things like "I searched and searched and tried and tried, and after years of struggling with failed diets and workouts, I finally found the secret!"

You buy their product or program. Maybe you use it. Maybe you don't. Chances are, you go full speed with it at first, like a hot new fling—but before long, it's back to square one. This weight loss "solution" fails to help you unearth the key to real change. It would be great if there were a magic pill you could swallow to have all you ever wanted and more, with no effort whatsoever. I'd be the first person in line to buy a big bottle. Hell, I'd buy two. Trust me, even with everything I know, I occasionally fall prey to this line of thinking, too.

It's time to wake up. You and I both know that transformation doesn't happen overnight.

Over the course of my life, I have found that the real key to unlocking your best body isn't some elaborate system of complex nutrition patterns and weird equipment-based workouts. The key is having a plan and acting on it *every day*.

Call it old-fashioned hard work, the kind of which our grandparents would be proud. Hey, it's vintage! Think about a farmer who wakes up every day before the sun rises and tends to the fields with great care. The success of her crop has a tremendous amount to do with elements that are completely out of her control, like the weather; but with a tenacity that we rarely see anymore, that farmer rolls up her sleeves and does the work (planting, tending, harvesting, and selling) that needs to be done in order to make a living. A successful farmer does this every day.

Now, before you throw this book out the window, I want to tell you something. Hard work doesn't need to be backbreaking. In fact, the work is made significantly easier if you have a decent plan—and oh, do I have a plan for you! Results are really more about consistency. Do the thing you need to do each day and before you know it—*bam!*—you're standing in the mirror asking, "Whose abs are *those*?"

If you read magazines and blogs or watch TV, you may see that I'm frequently called a "Celebrity Fitness Trainer" or "Wellness Guru"! Fancy schmancy, eh? Whatever. All I care about is helping you get where you want to be. I have spent considerable time, money, and effort over the course of twenty years to learn what works and what doesn't when it comes to fitness and, frankly, life in general. Do I have *all* the answers? Of course not. No one does. And anyone who says otherwise? Well, you should run as far away from them as possible. What I do know can help you cut your learning curve significantly and make life easier; techniques that took me years of trial and error to nail down are available to you in just a few pages. Consider this your ultimate playbook. I chose to publish in softcover for a reason: I want you to take it with you everywhere you go and really rough it up.

Eat Clean. Train Dirty. Live Hard. It's my mantra. It fuels my body, powers my workouts, and supercharges my life. Kind of rolls off the tongue, doesn't it? When I put that phrase on T-shirts and tanks, the inventory sells out in a few days. But as much as I love my mantra in its specific order, I'm switching that order in this book and leading with Train Dirty. Why? Because let's be honest, you bought this book for the wildly popular fitness plan responsible for those jaw-dropping before-and-after photos and all that buzz out there in the press. So in the spirit of making you super happy (see, I told you I care about you!), we're starting with Train Dirty. Then we'll dive into what it means to Eat Clean and Live Hard so you can see just how integral each part of that mantra is to losing weight fast and taking full control of your life.

Train Dirty lays out the six-week program I designed to help you torch fat, build long, lean muscle, and skyrocket your metabolism so that your body is burning calories even when you're not working out. It's fast, effective, and can be done anywhere, without a single piece of equipment. (See? I'm watching out for your wallet, too.)

In the second section, *Eat Clean,* I'll recommend a super-simple approach to eating that will totally change the way you think about the word *diet*. With this so-easy-you-won't-believe-it-works way to portion out your meals, you'll never need to count another calorie again. No weird and wacky gimmicks; just a sweet embrace of healthy, whole foods that are growing in a garden near you or available at your local grocery store. You'll feel good in your body and amazing in your soul knowing that you're making powerful yet remarkably simple choices that impact your waistline and your overall health: two-for-one!

In the third section, *Live Hard,* I'm going to teach you the best practices in self-development that will help you strengthen the single most important muscle in your body: your brain. I'm talking the crème de la crème: everything I've learned over the years, distilled to its most potent and straightforward essence. You'll learn how something I call Lottery Mindset Marketing has conditioned you to fail in your weight loss goals—and how to overcome it. You may actually find this to be the most valuable part of the entire book.

The tools in this book are just that: tools. If you don't use them, they will not work. This book will not give you flat abs through osmosis any more than a shovel is going to plant that apple tree for you. The power to achieve your fitness goals has always been, and will always be, inside of you.

You are the key. You are the vehicle. This book is your road map.

Let's put the pedal to the metal.

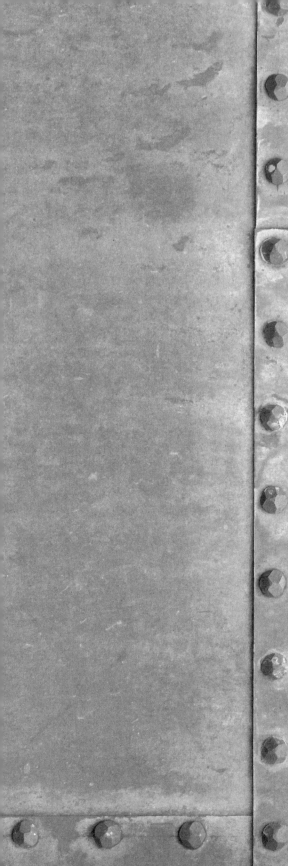
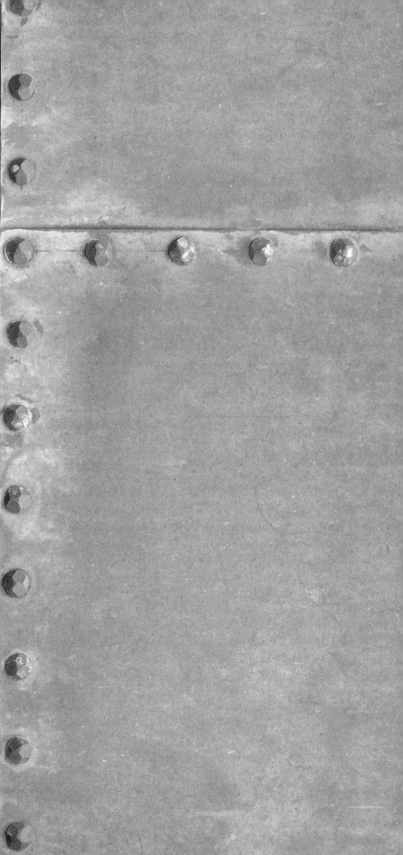

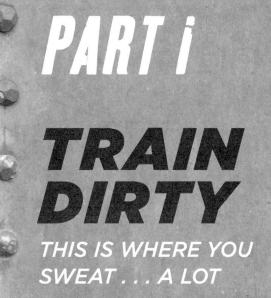

PART i

TRAIN DIRTY

THIS IS WHERE YOU
SWEAT . . . A LOT

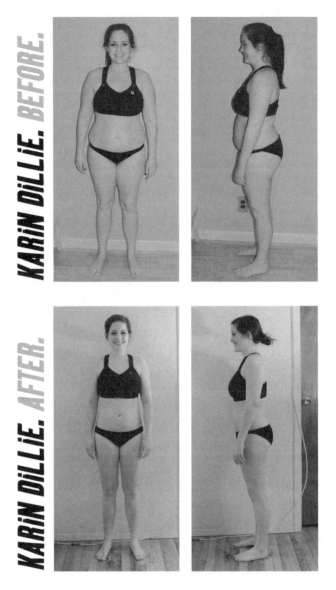

KARiN DiLLiE. BEFORE.

KARiN DiLLiE. AFTER.

"I did this challenge with a group of friends and I'll always remember after the very first workout when we were all a hot mess—soaked in sweat, hair all messed up, makeup everywhere—and we started to joke about how horrible we all looked. Not exactly the classic picture of 'sexy.' We believed that beauty came from things like exfoliating showers, mounds of hair spray, and perfect lip gloss. It wasn't until around week five, when I looked up during one of the more grueling exercises, that I finally started to see what Adam had seen in us since the beginning, what he sees in everyone—true strength. The kind of strength that comes from deep down within and emanates through every pore of our being. I saw that strength for what it was—real beauty. No diet or new fitness fad could give that to us. It was the product of working hard, eating real, whole food, and pushing ourselves past our perceived physical limits. It was the beauty that 30SB allowed us to find deep down within ourselves. And it sure was sexy."

WHAT THIS IS ALL ABOUT

ISN'T IT FUN SHUFFLING ALONG ON A TREAD-mill for an hour and a half? How about pounding it out on the pavement, mile after mile, till your knees ache and you miss happy hour with your friends? Don't forget about wandering around an overpriced, smelly gym trying to figure out how to use all the different machines. Doesn't that get you excited?

Yeah, I didn't think so. Doesn't do it for me, either. That's why I *train dirty*. It's a simple, no-nonsense, down-and-dirty approach to working out that takes far less time and is far more effective. You're not sitting pretty on some shiny machine giving a halfhearted effort while watching whatever's on the TV, only to walk away having barely raised your heart rate. No. You're *killing* it. When you're done, you're a hot, sweaty mess panting like a dog on a summer day. And it's a beautiful thing.

Back in the day, I used to work out just like most people. I'd mess around with weight machines, isolating single muscle groups for too long at a time—say, leg curls on one machine or seated shoulder presses on another—and then do a day of cardio where I ran for a while, usually on a treadmill. It wasn't ineffective, but it certainly wasn't revolutionary. Time, research, and practice eventually led me to discover the three foundational pillars of *The 30-Second Body,* which will light your workouts (and your body) on fire:

3

- Compound movements
- Progressive overload
- High-intensity intervals

You're not here to get a PhD in biomechanics; you're here to get in awesome shape, fast. So let's keep this simple.

Compound movements are exercises that incorporate multiple muscle groups at the same time. Compared to isolation exercises, like a single bicep curl, they are more efficient at elevating your heart rate, burning calories, and jacking up your metabolism. That all means a leaner, stronger body in less time. Compound movements also reflect the way the body naturally moves, as a whole, so you'll gain strength in a way that will help prevent injury over the long run. You know that friend of yours who looks like they're in really great shape, but pulled their back out moving a coffee table? This type of movement will help you *not* be that person. It's functional fitness. Think *strong for life*.

Progressive overload is the principle of challenging yourself to do a little more or a little better each time you work out. Whether that means an additional exercise, more reps, or even fewer reps with better form, when you constantly challenge your body, you constantly force it to grow. Practiced consistently, it will keep you in amazing shape forever. It sounds simple. And it is. But when you do it, it's radically effective.

High-intensity intervals means working out very intensely for periods of time (intervals) coupled with equal or slightly longer periods of lower-intensity work or full rest. This is the crown jewel. Many people have argued that doing long, slow cardio that keeps the body in a steady state (continuous, steady effort over a longer period of time) is better for fat loss. The rationale here is that the body uses a bit more fat as fuel during lower-intensity exercise than it does for higher intensities. If you remember or have ever heard of the "fat burning zone," this is what it's referring to; you're working at about 50 percent of your maximal heart rate. It's basically long, slow (read: boring) cardio. Think, mindlessly pumping along on the elliptical machine for an hour and change.

My version of high-intensity workouts presents a *much, much* better and more efficient way. Let me break it down:

Let's say you did 30 minutes of light cardio work where your heart rate was at 50 percent max. That will burn around 200 calories, with 120 of those coming from fat.

30 minutes. 200 total calories burned. 120 fat calories.

Now let's say you cranked up the heat and did 30 minutes of high-intensity work where your heart rate was around 75 percent max. That will burn about 400 calories, of which 140 will come from fat.

30 minutes. 400 total calories. 140 fat calories.

See the difference?

You burn more fat at high intensities than you do at low intensities. And it takes less time to burn more. Any reason you'd *not* want to lose more weight in less time? Also, this type of training ignites the "afterburn effect." Sounds schmancy, but again, it's really simple. It means your body continues to burn calories after your workout is over. Yup! That's right; while you're sitting on your butt, your metabolism is like a little ninja, slicing and dicing calories like crazy. To explain this a bit further, you'll increase your resting metabolic rate (the amount of calories your body burns while at rest) for up to 38 hours *after* a high-intensity workout. Here's why: The more intensely you work out, the more oxygen your body consumes afterward. That sustains your metabolic rate at a higher level, which means you're burning more calories. Light cardio burns almost no calories post-exercise; it only does so *at the time* one is engaged in it.

Let's be clear: I'm not saying that there is no benefit to steady-state cardio. I think we can all agree that moving the body in *any* way is a good thing. It's also great to mix things up. Plus, some people who try to go too fast too soon may abandon exercise completely, as it's too much of a shock to their bodies. It's important to know where you are and proceed accordingly, at the level that is most comfortable for you. In part, that's the beauty of the workouts I'm giving you here. Going for time, not reps, which is exactly what you're going to do, will allow you to work at your own pace and progress from there, getting stronger and faster with each session. That slow, boring cardio *will* lead to weight loss; it's just going to take longer.

So, if you want to get in great shape fast, you need to pump up the volume with some high-intensity training.

PUTTING THE PIECES TOGETHER

OKAY, LET'S ASSEMBLE THIS. WITH MY WORK-outs you're going to be doing compound movements that bring on progressive overload and you'll be doing them at a high intensity for intervals of time (30 seconds per movement for the first two weeks; we kick it up to 60 in the last two weeks—remember the law of progressive overload?). There are no weights or equipment, so you can do these workouts anywhere, anytime. Your living room, basement, backyard, a nearby park, a beach in the Caribbean—anywhere you can carve out a few feet of space is your training center to lose a ton of weight and tone up every inch of your body.

I've also organized your workouts neatly into a little calendar so that you can check days off as you go (there's something *so* grati-fying about that, isn't there?). Each of your first two weeks of work-outs lasts less than 25 minutes from start to finish, and I've also thrown in a few 5-Minute Quick Fire sessions. So if for some reason you can't get in a full workout, you can rock one of these bad boys and have at least done something.

Full disclosure: I ran my mom through a 5-Minute Quick Fire

and she was huffing for breath wondering how this short routine could be more strenuous than her hour-plus class at the gym. And if you have more than five minutes, but less than twenty-five, you can stack a few of these or just repeat the circuit as your time allows.

Ready to unlock your best body? Here are your next steps:

#1 *Get Cleared for Exercise*

This may sound silly, but I'm serious. Before you begin any exercise program, you need to check with your doctor to be sure there are no undiscovered issues that would prevent you from diving into an intense workout regimen. I'm not trying to be an alarmist or cover my butt here. My number-one concern is for your health and well-being. Please, go see the doc and make sure you're good to go.

#2 *Pledge to Lose*

You're the one in charge here. All I'm doing is providing you with the guidance you need to get in the best shape of your life. But if you don't stay committed, this simply will not work. I've found that having my clients sign a pledge helps them stay on track. This isn't a pledge to me. It's a contract with yourself. Sign it and stick it on your fridge as a reminder of your commitment to live a healthy, active life.

> On this date, _____, 20____, I promise to take control of my health and happiness by starting and completing the 30-Second Body 6-Week Challenge. When I smile at myself in the mirror six

weeks from now, on this date, _____, 20____, I'll think back on this moment with pride. Starting right now, I pledge to:

CARE for my body and mind with great food, exercise, and sleep.

BELIEVE in my ability to do my personal best and tap my inner strength to power through the difficult times.

KNOW that there will be difficult times, but that I am capable of anything.

UNDERSTAND there are no magic pills or shortcuts, only my commitment to doing the work and belief in my ability to achieve my goals.

LOVE myself as I am *right now*.

ENJOY this process. Life is meant to be fun!

I know that as I exist right now, I am perfect. This 6-Week Challenge is simply going to enhance that. Fear, shame, and guilt are no longer emotions that I will allow to hold me back. I am fully in charge of my life!

_____   _____
Signature   Date

#3 Recruit Your Crew

You can definitely take this journey on your own. But it's a lot easier and a whole lot more fun to stay committed with a community. You'll become a source of inspiration and motivation for one another. And you can share recipes and stories, and curse me out together! Plus, taking this journey with other people helps hold you accountable. So tap a few peeps you think would be down with six weeks of sweat-dripping transformational fun and dive into this together. You may even want to surprise them by picking up a copy of this book for them. It's hard to say no to something when you've just been presented with a gift, you sneaky little devil, you!

#4 *Snap Some Pics. Take Some Measurements.*

I want you to take pictures of yourself and measurements on three different days during this process. The scale can be confusing. From muscle tone to water retention, there are so many factors that affect that silly number. Step on the scale if you'd like, but I want you to be empowered and motivated both by visual proof and the strength and health you'll feel in your body.

On a day-to-day basis, we don't always notice positive changes, but I promise they add up. If you don't have the pictures or measurements, you'll regret not documenting your amazing transformation.

Have a friend or family member take the photos if you'd like (another benefit of doing this challenge with friends). If you'd prefer to do it on your own, just use a mirror.

Change into a bathing suit and snap the following pics on the following days:

- Frontal
- Profile (left and right)
- Rear (shoot over your shoulder if you're doing it alone)
- Take all the pics on Day 1 and again at the end of Weeks 3 and 6

For the measurements, you'll need a cloth measuring tape (the kind a tailor uses). Some of these are a lot easier if you have someone else doing the measuring. Make sure to keep the tape level and snug, neither tight nor loose. Measure over bare skin and be sure that you are measuring in the exact same spot each time. Last, write your measurements down on the chart below:

DATE	Day 1	End of Week 3	End of Week 6
Left Bicep Halfway between your shoulder and elbow			
Right Bicep Same as above			
Chest Right across the nipples. Be sure to put your arms by your sides so you're getting the true measurement of your back as well.			
Waist Right across the belly button			
Hips Stand with legs and feet together. Measure across the widest part of your butt.			
Left Thigh Stand with feet shoulder-width apart. Measure your thigh halfway between your inseam and knee.			
Right Thigh Same as above			
Left Calf Measure across the thickest part of your calf			
Right Calf Same as above			

#5 Build a Strong Foundation

All the moves in your workouts are based on a series of functional, foundational movements. It's REALLY IMPORTANT (sorry to shout, but really, this is important) that you pay careful attention to your form. Sloppy form leads to injuries, so take some time to practice these moves first, going nice and slow to ensure you're doing them correctly.

- Squat
- Lunge
- Push-up
- Jump

SQUAT

Stand with your feet shoulder-width apart, toes turned out slightly, arms relaxed by your side. Open your chest and pull your shoulder blades down your back. Engage your core, as this will help stabilize your spine. Think of pulling your belly button in and up, then squeezing your abs nice and tight. Keep your chest lifted and chin parallel to the floor as you inhale and push your hips back to lower down until upper thighs are at least parallel to the ground (think of this as trying to sit down in a chair that someone's pulling out from under you). Lower down as far as you can without losing the natural curve in your lower back. The weight should be mostly on your heels. Exhale as you push into your heels and return to start. Squeeze your butt at the top of the movement.

LUNGE

Stand with feet together. Open your chest, pull your shoulder blades down your back, and engage your core. Maintaining a straight back, step forward with one foot to land heel first. Shift your body weight to the lead foot and drop the hips straight down until the front thigh is parallel to the floor, being sure to keep the front knee behind the toes. Push off the front leg and return to the starting position. Repeat with the opposite leg.

PUSH-UP

Start on your hands and knees with wrists directly below the shoulders. Open your chest, pull your shoulder blades down your back, and engage your core. Step back, one leg at a time, to the top of a push-up position. Keep your neck aligned with your spine and slowly bend the elbows straight back toward the feet to lower your body to 1 inch above the floor. Do not allow your back to sag or hips to pike. Maintaining a rigid torso and keeping your neck in line with your spine, press back up to the starting position.

* If you can't perform a full-range-of-motion push-up with proper form (all the way to the floor and up again without sagging or piking the hips), perform your push-ups from your knees until you've built the strength to step back. Warning: DO NOT CALL THESE "GIRL" PUSH-UPS! I will hunt you down.

JUMP

Stand with your feet hip-width apart, arms relaxed by your side. Open your chest, pull your shoulder blades down your back, and engage your core. Push your hips back and down to lower yourself until your thighs are parallel to the floor. Maintain a flat back, and keep your head facing forward. Your arms should be in front of you (like you're about to catch a football) to offer maximum balance. Pause very briefly at the bottom of the downward phase and explode up, fully extending your hips, knees, and ankles as you swing your arms backward. As you jump, keep your feet level with each other and parallel to the floor. Land softly on the mid-foot and roll to the heels as you push your hips back and down to absorb the impact. **Never land with locked knees!**

* You can watch free videos of each of these moves at www.the30secondbody .com.

#6 *Do Your First Fit Test. Write Down Your Results.*

Your fit test is a challenge comprising six moves that will assess your baseline fitness level. In the *Get Fit Fast Tools* section, beginning on page 19, you'll find a tracking grid where you'll log your results as well as descriptions for each of the moves. You'll do each move for 60 seconds, trying to get as many reps as possible while maintaining perfect form. You can also print this out for free at www.the30secondbody.com.

#7 *Check Your Calendar*

In your *Get Fit Fast Tools* section below, you'll find a complete calendar with all of your workouts for the full six weeks. Take a minute to look it over and get acquainted with the layout. This is also available as a free printout at www.the30secondbody.com.

#8 *Start the Challenge!*

Your plan consists of five workouts each week, plus a day of Recovery Yoga for a total of six weeks. They're outlined and broken out in detail with photos and instructions in *The Workouts* section below.

Break It Up and Reward Yourself

Instead of looking at this program as one big six-week challenge, think of it as three two-week periods. It's a small shift in mindset that can make all this so much more doable.

And do you know what motivates almost as much as results?

Treats! At the end of each two-week period, reward yourself with a little something. That pair of sneakers you've been eyeing, a new workout top, a massage, some new bath salts, whatever makes sense for you and your budget.

Just make sure it's a healthy gift (no getting wasted or crappy food as a reward!) and you'll be so much more likely to stay in the game and push even harder toward those end-of-week markers.

#9 Check In on Weeks 3 and 6

Speaking of being motivated by results, at the end of weeks 3 and 6 you're going to take your photos and measurements again. Be proud of the work you've been doing up to each of these points. It may not be easy, but just wait till you discover how amazing you can feel and what your body is capable of achieving.

Gear and Other Stuff

All of these workouts are equipment-free. That said, there are a few things that can enhance your experience.

- **Sneakers**—A pair that provides proper cushion and support. While the workouts can be done barefoot, if you're not maintaining proper form it will be much easier for you to get injured. So don't cheap out; use the money you'll save on the gym for a good pair of kicks. Cross-trainers are great and some brands make sneakers that are designed specifically for high-intensity interval training.
- **Interval Timer**—This is really critical. There is no way you'll be

able to keep proper time with a stopwatch or clock on the wall. You can download one of the many free apps that are out there, buy yourself a Gymboss timer, or get a wristwatch with an interval timer function. I use one called the Timex Ironman Triathlon for my personal workouts, private sessions, and group classes, but any interval timer will tick off the workout time and then reset itself without your having to do a thing. Find one you like and get it today.

- **Music**—This is such a key feature in my classes and workouts. Generally speaking, the higher the tempo, the more intense the workout, but just pick whatever really gets you going.

- **Extra Cushion**—If you're doing your workouts on a hard surface, such as in a carpeted basement, the impact can be really hard on your joints. Pick up a thick exercise mat like my Impact Plyo Mat, available at www.the30secondbody.com. *Never* perform these workouts on a concrete or pavement surface.

- **Muscle Relief**—You're going to get sore. That's not a bad thing! You can ice the sore area, take Epsom salt baths, and/or hit the sauna and steam room.

- **Foam Roller**—This technically could fall under Muscle Relief or Recovery, but I think it deserves its own bullet point! Foam rolling is one of the best ways to keep your muscles loose and your body mobile. My fave is the Trigger Point Therapy Grid Foam Roller. You can get it online or at most sporting goods stores. It's small and can fit in the corner of your closet and even comes with simple picture instructions. There are also these wonderful things called Yoga Tune Up balls. Amazing and highly portable, they get in there in a way a foam roller just can't! Whether it's the balls or the roller, get one and use it daily!

- **Recovery**—Post-workout protein intake will help improve your recovery and results. Within 45 minutes of completing your workout, have a protein shake. It could be as simple as a powder protein mixed with water, or you can add a banana or other fruit and blend it all up if you'd like.

- **Water**—These workouts are going to make you sweat. Make sure you're properly hydrated before starting and that you have a bottle of water on hand during your sessions. Drink up after.

- **Sleep**—I can't stress this enough: A world of magical restoration occurs while we're sleeping. So please, make sure you're getting 7–8 hours of quality sleep every night.

Matt Stueland, 37, Media Executive

Results: Lost 2 inches. 20 percent decrease in cholesterol.

I wasn't one of those guys who needed to lose a huge amount of weight, but I always wanted to actually see my abs. To be honest, it always felt like a never-ending road. Adam's program made it happen. My results were unparalleled to any diet or workout regimen I had tried in the past. In two months, working out only two times per week, I lost two inches! But what's really crazy is the completely unexpected result that I got from the program, which affected something far more serious than how I look in a bathing suit.

I come from a family history of high cholesterol and, after years of being monitored by my doctor, was on the verge of going on medication (which I did not want to do since I'm still in my thirties). No matter what I did, my levels consistently remained between 220 and 240. In September and November 2012 my total cholesterol levels were 239 and 237 despite maintaining a healthy diet and a couple of days of cardio each week. In February 2013, again, only *two months* after training on Adam's program *only two days per week*, my total cholesterol dropped over 20 percent, to 187! My dangerous LDL levels went from 160 to 117 (my lowest LDL prior to this was 133). I was blown away. Adam is simply the best of the best. Anyone who has a chance to follow his program should consider themselves blessed—it will not only make you stronger physically, it'll raise your mental toughness and reveal the possibilities of how much you can accomplish in all aspects of your life. And it definitely doesn't hurt that I look damn good in a bathing suit now.

GET FiT FAST TOOLS

IN THIS SECTION, YOU'LL GET YOUR FIT TEST along with instructions for those moves, explanations of the warm-up routine, the three workouts plus a recovery yoga routine, and the cooldown process. I will also give you a complete 6-Week Workout Calendar (also reprinted at the back of the book so you can tear it out and post it on your wall if that's the way you roll).

Fit Test

Perform each exercise for 60 seconds, trying to get as many reps as possible while maintaining perfect form. This is where that interval timer is going to first come into play.

Keep track of your reps as you're doing them. Write them down after each exercise.

Rest 30 seconds between moves.

Exercise	Fit Test 1	Fit Test 2	Fit Test 3
Tuck Jumps			
Push-ups			
Pencil Squats Return to standing position = 1 rep			
3-Point Plankers Feet come center = 1 rep			
Standing Mountain Climbers 2 knees = 1 rep			
Power Thrusts			

* Available as a printout at www.the30secondbody.com.

FIT TEST MOVE INSTRUCTIONS

Tuck Jump

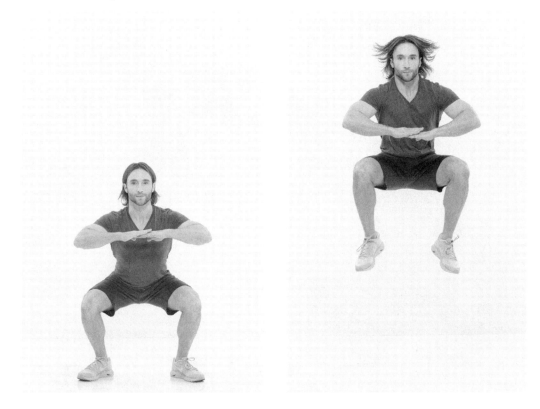

Stand with your feet shoulder-width apart, arms at a T at chest level with fingers interlaced or stacked. Press the hips back into a squat and immediately explode upward, driving the knees toward the forearms. Land softly and quietly on the mid-foot, rolling back to the heels. Immediately push the hips back to absorb the impact of the landing. Repeat.

* **Modification:** Lose the jump. Perform a squat as indicated above. At the top of the motion, raise the right knee to the forearm and lower the foot to the floor. Perform another squat repeating the leg movement on the other side. That's 1 rep.

Push-ups

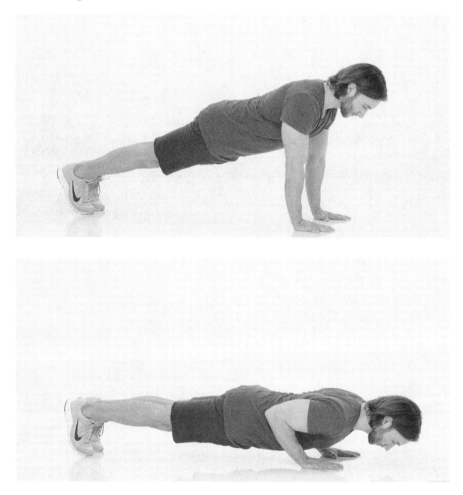

Start in the top of a push-up position with your wrists directly below your shoulders. Brace your core and pull your shoulder blades down your back. Bend the elbows straight back, keeping them close to your sides, to lower your body to the floor. Come to 1 inch above the floor and press upward through your arms to straighten the elbows. Make sure to keep your head in line with your spine and your torso straight throughout the entire movement. Repeat.

* **Modification:** Drop knees to floor, keeping them behind the hips.

Pencil Squats

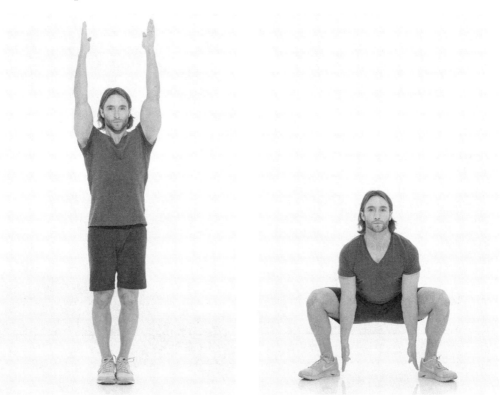

Stand with your feet together, arms raised overhead. Hop your feet apart to drop down into a low squat while reaching the fingertips down behind your heels. Keep your chest up and your back neutral at the bottom of the movement. Explosively return to the starting position. Repeat.

* **Modification:** Lose the hops. Step out to the right, lower into a squat, and back to start. Repeat on opposite side. Arm movements are the same.

3-Point Plankers

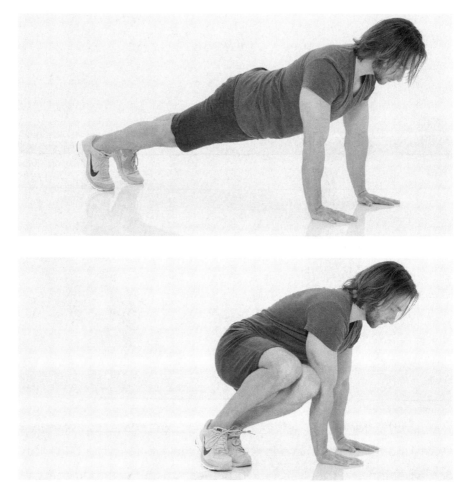

Assume a push-up position. Keep the hands flat on the floor with wrists under shoulders and jump the feet as close as you can to the outside of the left hand. Return to start. Jump the feet as close as you can to the outside of the right hand. Return to start. Now jump the feet between the hands. Return to start. That's 1 rep. Continue repeating the move.

* **Modification:** Step the feet, one at a time, toward the hands and back.

Standing Mountain Climbers

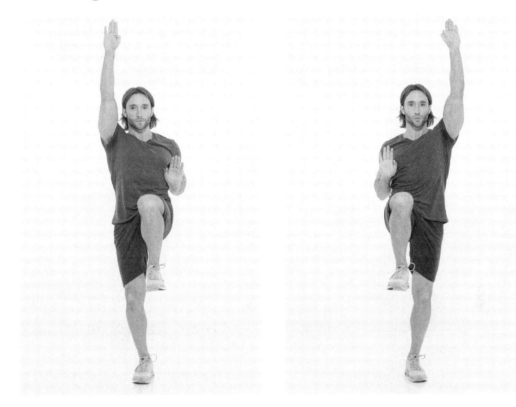

Stand with feet hip-width apart and hands in front of shoulders, palms facing forward. Brace your core and pull your shoulder blades down your back. Shoot your right fingertips to the sky as you raise your left knee up to hip height. Explosively switch sides, shooting the left fingertips to the sky as you raise your right knee to hip height. Continue alternating.

* **Modification:** Lose the explosive switch and simply alternate knee lifts while reaching the arms overhead.

Power Thrusts

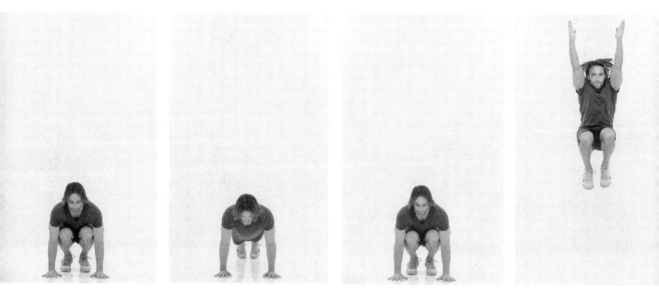

Stand with feet wider than hip-width apart. Squat down and place your hands on the floor, wrists positioned under your shoulders. Kick your feet back so that you're at the top of a push-up position. Immediately return them to the squat position. Explosively jump up off the floor, shooting your fingertips to the sky and driving your knees high up toward your chest. Land softly and quietly on the mid-foot, rolling back to the heels. Immediately push the hips back to absorb the impact of the landing. Repeat.

* **Modification:** Don't kick the feet back. Step back and then forward, one foot at a time. At the top of the movement, lose the jump and bring one knee at a time up to hip height with arms raised overhead.

The Warm-up

You're going to do this dynamic warm-up before every workout with the exception of *Recovery Yoga*. Warming up dynamically is the best way to prepare your body for exercise and help prevent injury.

This specific warm-up is one that I designed to progressively activate every muscle and joint in your body. Start slowly and gradually pick up the pace for each move, going at your own pace. When you get more advanced, you should almost be in a full sprint during the high knees.

The warm-up is 100 percent necessary. Please, never skip it.

Move	Time
• To be performed before every workout (*except Recovery Yoga*). • Keep your core engaged for every move.	
Forward Shoulder Rolls Stand with feet hip-width apart, chest open, shoulders pulled down your back, and core engaged. Keep the neck long and head high as you roll the shoulders forward. Get a nice full range of motion.	**10 seconds**
Reverse Shoulder Rolls Same as above, but reversed.	**10 seconds**
Forward March-in-Place Windmills March in place as you sweep the arms forward in large circles. Keep leg movement and arm movement in sync. Arms come up, leg comes up. Arms come down, leg comes down.	**10 seconds**
Reverse March-in-Place Windmills Same as above, but arms are going backward and the legs are each coming straight up and back in a reverse circular motion.	**10 seconds**
Chest Openers Stand with feet hip-width apart. Keep the neck long and head high as you reach the fingertips forward. Draw your shoulders back and down. Open the left arm out to the side, in line with the shoulder, and back to the front. Repeat on the right. Make sure to keep your arms parallel to the floor. Continue alternating.	**10 seconds**

Move	Time
Twisting Takedowns Stand with the feet wider than hip-width, arms extended out to the side. Twist the torso to the left and then take the left fingertips down to the outside of the right foot. Return to center. Twist the torso to the right and then take the right fingertips down to the outside of the left foot. Return to center. Continue alternating. This one takes a little coordination so don't get frustrated if it takes you a few tries to get it right!	**10 seconds**
Jumping Jacks Touch your fingers at the top and slap your thighs lightly at the bottom. Keep toes and knees in line with one another.	**10 seconds**
Crossover Jacks Stand with the feet wider than hip width, arms extended out to the side. Cross the right arm over the left as you simultaneously jump the right leg over the left. Return to center. Repeat on the opposite side. Continue alternating.	**10 seconds**
Lateral Jumps Stand with feet hip-width apart, knees bent, hips slightly back. Jump side to side over an imaginary line bringing the knees up to hip height.	**10 seconds**
Butt Kicks Jog in place, bringing each heel up to kick yourself lightly in the butt. Keep your hips forward and knees close together.	**20 seconds**
High Knees Extend arms forward parallel to the floor and hold there. Run in place, bringing each knee up toward elbows. 1 rep = left knee and right knee.	**20 seconds**

CARDiO BLAZE

This is a high-intensity workout that torches fat by keeping you moving with speed and precision.

Exercise	Time Duration

- Perform the first four moves back-to-back for the instructed time, with as little rest as possible during and between moves.
- Once you've finished all four moves, that's the end of Round 1.
- Rest 30 seconds and repeat, this time adding the fifth move. That's the end of Round 2.
- Rest another 30 seconds and repeat, this time adding the sixth move. That's the end of Round 3.
- Do not stop the timer.

Exercise	Time Duration
High Knee Jump Rope	**30 seconds (Weeks 1–3)** 60 seconds (Weeks 4-6)
Tuck Jumps	**30 seconds (Weeks 1–3)** 60 seconds (Weeks 4-6)
Mountain Terrainers	**30 seconds (Weeks 1–3)** 60 seconds (Weeks 4-6)
Standing Mountain Climbers	**30 seconds (Weeks 1–3)** 60 seconds (Weeks 4-6)
Low Plank Knees (add to end of Round 2)	**30 seconds (Weeks 1–3)** 60 seconds (Weeks 4-6)
High Plank Punches (add to end of Round 3, after Low Plank Knee-ins)	**30 seconds (Weeks 1–3)** 60 seconds (Weeks 4-6)

HEAT 1

- Once you've completed Round 3, rest 30 seconds and move on to Heat 2 in the same format as above.
- The only difference with Heat 2 is that at the end of Round 3 you're immediately going to perform the 100 Meter Dash as a seventh move.

Exercise	Time Duration
Pencil Squats	**30 seconds (Weeks 1–3)** 60 seconds (Weeks 4-6)
Oblique High Knees	**30 seconds (Weeks 1–3)** 60 seconds (Weeks 4-6)
Spiders	**30 seconds (Weeks 1–3)** 60 seconds (Weeks 4-6)
3-Point Plankers	**30 seconds (Weeks 1–3)** 60 seconds (Weeks 4-6)
Low Squat Sprints (add to end of Round 2)	**30 seconds (Weeks 1–3)** 60 seconds (Weeks 4-6)
Power Thrusts (add to end of Round 3)	**30 seconds (Weeks 1–3)** 60 seconds (Weeks 4-6)
100-Meter Dash (add to end of Round 3, after Power Thrusts)	**30 seconds (Weeks 1–3)** 60 seconds (Weeks 4-6)

• Rest 1 minute. Do your Cool Down.

HEAT 2

High Knee Jump Rope

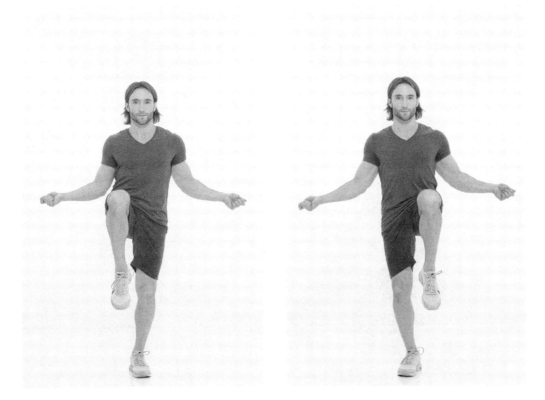

While swinging an imaginary jump rope, sprint in place as fast as you can, raising knees to hip level. Sync the rope with your skips. Continue alternating.

Tuck Jumps

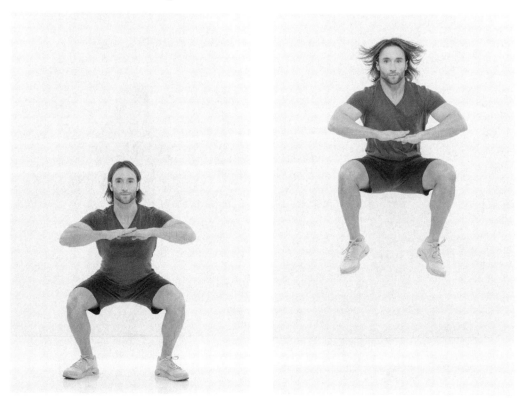

Stand with your feet shoulder-width apart, arms at a T at chest level with fingers interlaced or stacked. Press the hips back into a squat and immediately explode upward, driving the knees toward the forearms. Land softly and quietly on the mid-foot, rolling back to the heels. Immediately push the hips back to absorb the impact of the landing. Repeat.

* **Modification:** Lose the jump. Perform a squat as indicated above. At the top of the motion, raise the right knee to the forearm and lower the foot to the floor. Perform another squat, repeating the leg movement on the other side.

Mountain Terrainers

This is a combo move consisting of four standard Mountain Climbers and four X-Body Mountain Climbers.

MOUNTAIN CLIMBERS

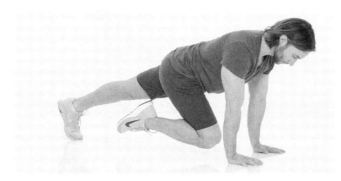

Assume a push-up position. Brace the core and bring the right knee toward the chest. Return to start as you bring the left knee toward the chest. That's 1 rep. Continue alternating.

X-BODY MOUNTAIN CLIMBERS

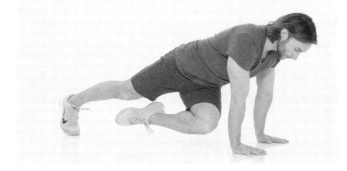

Assume a push-up position. Bring the left knee across the body toward the right elbow. Return to start as you bring the right knee across the body toward the left elbow. Return to start. That's 1 rep. Continue alternating.

Standing Mountain Climbers

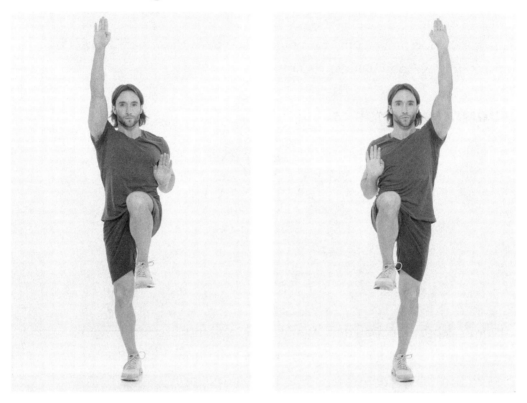

Stand with feet hip-width apart and hands in front of shoulders, palms facing forward. Brace your core and pull your shoulder blades down your back. Shoot your right fingertips to the sky as you raise your left knee up to hip height. Explosively switch sides, shooting the left fingertips to the sky as you raise your right knee to hip height. Continue alternating.

Low Plank Knees

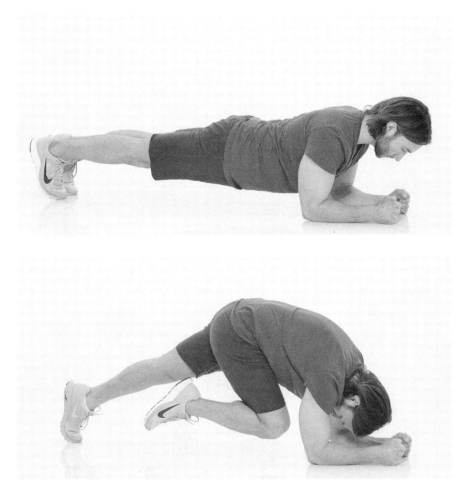

Assume a low plank position, forearms on the floor with elbows directly below shoulders. You should have a perfectly straight line from head to heels. Brace your core and pike your hips as you drive your right knee toward your face and return to start. Repeat the motion on the opposite side. Continue alternating. Be sure to lower your hips all the way back to start after each rep.

High Plank Punches

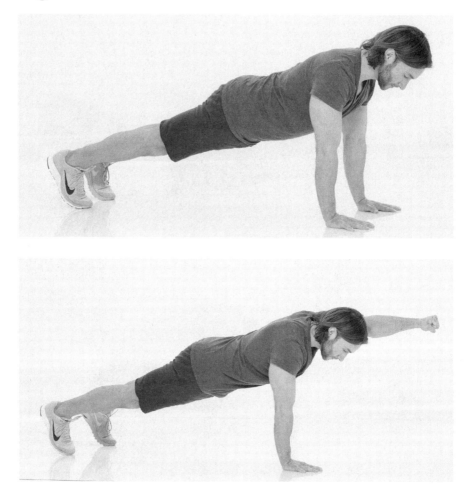

Assume a push-up position with wrists directly under shoulders. Punch forward with the left fist at shoulder level. Place hand back on floor. Repeat with the right fist.

Pencil Squats

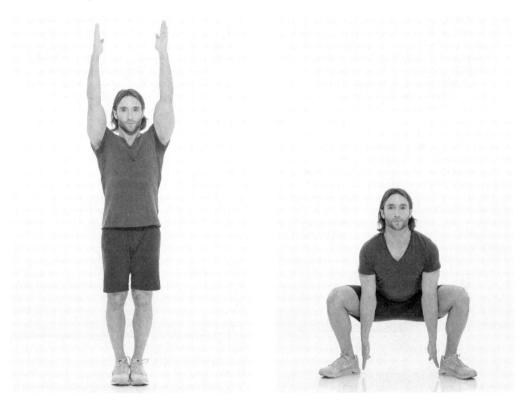

Stand with your feet together, arms raised overhead at shoulder width. Hop the feet apart to drop down into a low squat and touch the floor just behind your ankles. Explosively return to the starting position. Repeat.

* **Modification:** Lose the hops. Step out to the right, lower into a squat, and back to start. Arm movements are the same.

Oblique High Knees

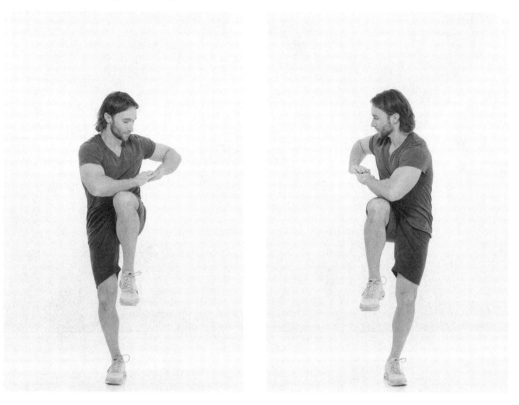

Stand tall with your feet shoulder-width apart and arms forming a T at chest level. Sprint in place, raising knees to hip height while bringing opposite elbows toward opposite knees.

Spiders

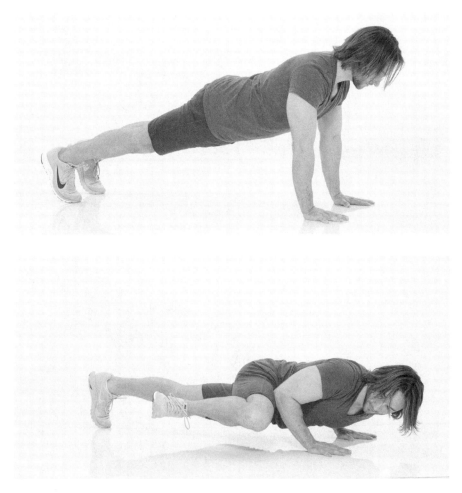

Assume a push-up position with wrists directly under the shoulders. Bend the elbows straight back to lower the chest to 1 inch above the floor. As you lower, bring the right knee in toward the right elbow. Press back up to start. Repeat the motion with the left knee. That's 1 rep.

* **Modification:** Perform the move with your knees on the floor. To further modify, perform regular push-ups.

3-Point Plankers

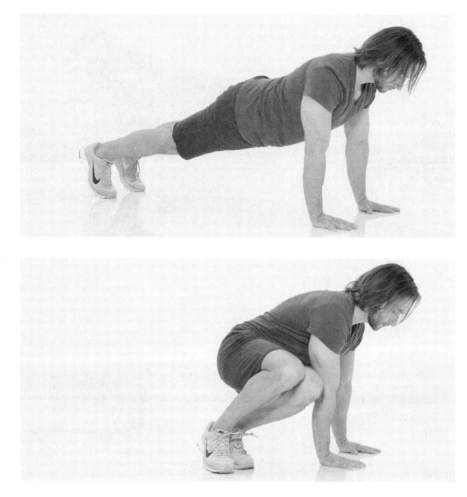

Assume a push-up position. Keep the hands flat on the floor and jump the feet as close as you can to the outside of the right hand. Return to start. Jump the feet as close as you can to the outside of the left hand. Return to start. Now jump the feet between the hands. Return to start. That's 1 rep. Continue repeating the move.

* **Modification:** Step the feet, one at a time, toward the hands and back, one at a time, to start.

Low Squat Sprints

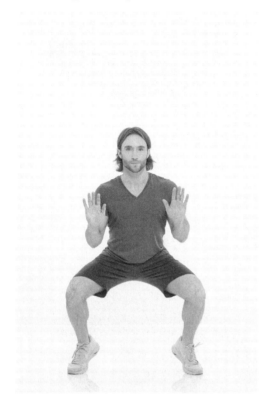

Start in a low squat with hips pressed back to at least knee level. Keep your chest up and chin parallel to the floor with your hands raised to chest level (as if you were going to stop someone from running into you). Raise up to the balls of your feet and sprint in place as fast as you can while alternately pumping the hands forward.

Power Thrusts

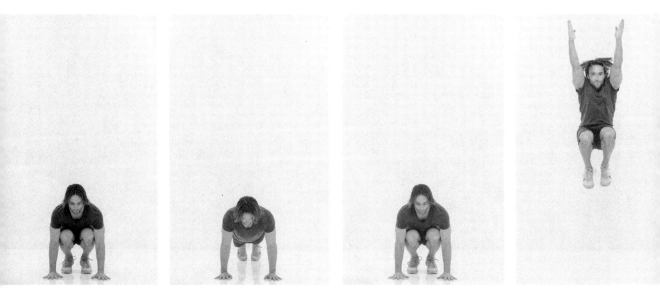

Stand with feet wider than hip-width apart. Squat down and place your hands on the floor, wrists positioned under your shoulders. Kick your feet back so that you're at the top of a push-up position. Immediately return them to the squat position. Explosively jump up off the floor, shooting your fingertips to the sky and driving your knees high up toward your chest. Land softly and quietly on the mid-foot, rolling back to the heels. Immediately push the hips back to absorb the impact of the landing. Repeat.

* **Modification:** Don't kick the feet back. Step back and then forward, one foot at a time. At the top of the movement, lose the jump and bring one knee at a time up to hip height with arms raised overhead.

100-Meter Dash

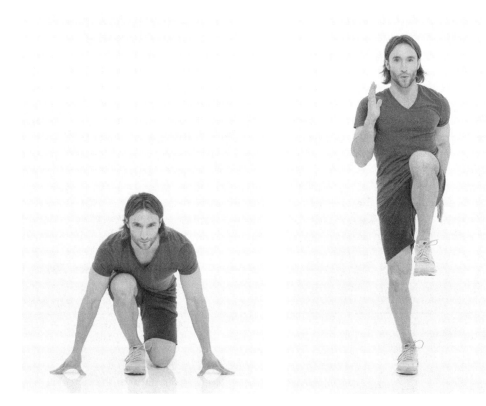

Sprint in place as fast as you can, pumping your arms and raising your knees to at least hip level.

* **Modification:** Slow down.

AiRBORNE

This is a plyometric-based workout that uses explosive jumping movements to build lean muscle and explosive power.

Exercise	Time Duration

- Perform the first four moves back-to-back for the instructed time, with as little rest as possible during and between moves.
- Once you've finished all four moves, that's the end of Round 1.
- Rest 30 seconds and repeat, this time adding the fifth move. That's the end of Round 2.
- Rest another 30 seconds and repeat, this time adding the sixth move. That's the end of Round 3.
- Do not stop the timer.

Exercise	Time Duration
180s	**30 seconds (Weeks 1–3)** 60 seconds (Weeks 4–6)
Ladder Climbers	**30 seconds (Weeks 1–3)** 60 seconds (Weeks 4–6)
Tap-ups	**30 seconds (Weeks 1–3)** 60 seconds (Weeks 4–6)
Starbursts	**30 seconds (Weeks 1–3)** 60 seconds (Weeks 4–6)
Power Kicks	**30 seconds (Weeks 1–3)** 60 seconds (Weeks 4–6)
High Lows	**30 seconds (Weeks 1–3)** 60 seconds (Weeks 4–6)

HEAT 1

- Once you've completed Round 3, rest 30 seconds, then move on to Heat 2 in the same format as above.
- The only difference with Heat 2 is that at the end of Round 3 you're immediately going to perform the 100 Meter Dash as a seventh move.

Exercise	Time Duration
Plié Jumps	**30 seconds (Weeks 1–3)** 60 seconds (Weeks 4–6)
Squat Push-ups	**30 seconds (Weeks 1–3)** 60 seconds (Weeks 4–6)
Deep Mountain Climbers	**30 seconds (Weeks 1–3)** 60 seconds (Weeks 4–6)
Long-Jump Sprints	**30 seconds (Weeks 1–3)** 60 seconds (Weeks 4–6)
Table Saws (add to end of Round 2)	**30 seconds (Weeks 1–3)** 60 seconds (Weeks 4–6)
Laterals (add to the end of Round 3, after Table Saws)	**30 seconds (Weeks 1–3)** 60 seconds (Weeks 4–6)
100-Meter Dash (add to end of Round 3, after Laterals)	**30 seconds (Weeks 1–3)** 60 seconds (Weeks 4–6)

• Rest 1 minute. Do your Cool Down.

HEAT 2

180s

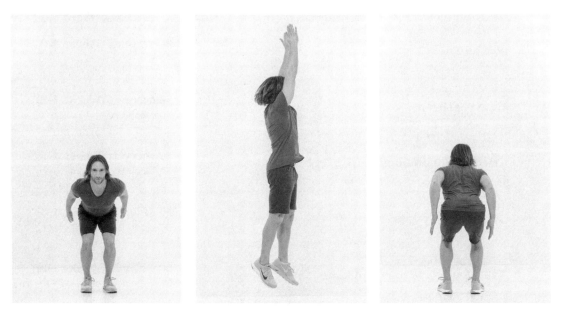

Stand with your feet hip-width apart, arms by your sides. Push your hips back as you bring your hands in front of you in a jump prep position. Explosively jump up off the floor and rotate 180 degrees in the air to land softly in the opposite direction. Repeat, turning back to face the starting direction.

* **Modification:** Lose the jump. Perform a squat. At the top of the motion, pivot on the ball of the right foot and swing your body around 180 degrees. Repeat, coming back to start.

Ladder Climbers

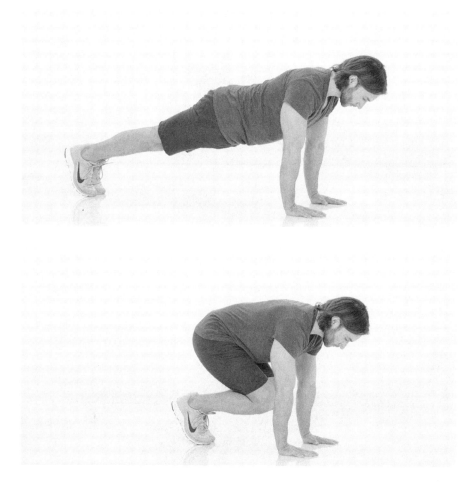

Assume a push-up position. Imagine that your body is above a ladder with your hands on the outsides of it and your feet at the bottom. Keep your hands flat on the floor, brace your core, and jump the feet forward about 1 foot, as if you were jumping them into the first box of the ladder. Return to start. Jump the feet forward about 2 feet, as if into the second box of the ladder. Return to start. Now jump the feet close to the hands, as if into the third box of the ladder. Jump the feet back to start. Continue repeating.

* **Modification:** Step the feet forward and then back, one foot at a time.

Tap-ups

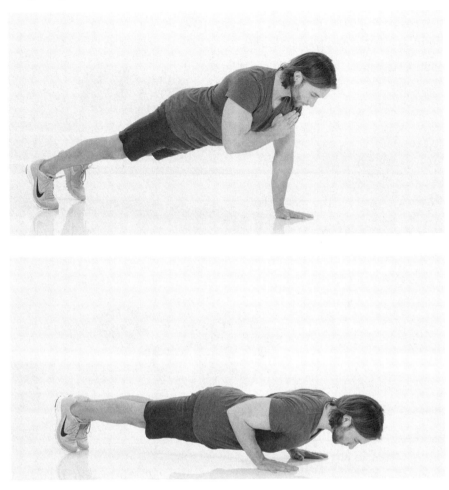

Assume a push-up position. Tap the left shoulder with right finger-tips and return the hand to the floor. Tap the right shoulder with the left fingertips and return the hand to the floor. Perform a push-up. Repeat.

Starbursts

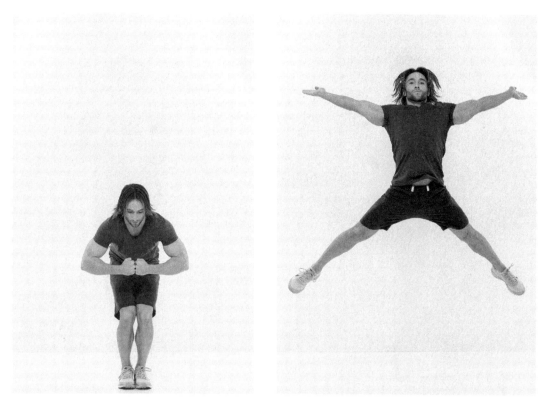

Stand with feet together. Bend the knees and push the hips back into a low squat, contracting your core and drawing your arms in to the center of your body. Pause only briefly at the bottom of the movement and explosively jump up as high as you can, extending arms and legs out to form an X. Land softly and repeat.

* **Modification:** Lose the jump. Squat low and stand, extending arms overhead into a Y and right leg out to form half an X. Repeat with opposite leg.

Power Kicks

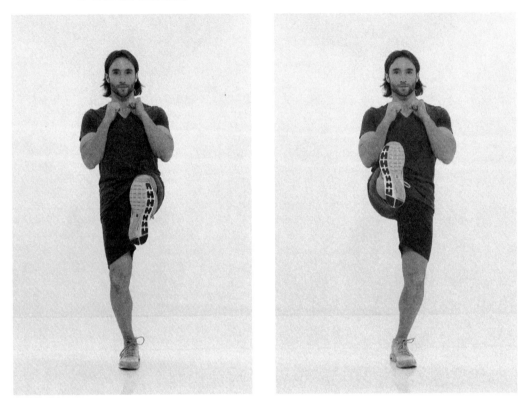

Stand with your feet slightly wider than hip-width apart, fists clenched just below your chin. Kick forward with your left foot up to at least hip level, extending through the heel. Explosively switch feet, lowering the left foot as you kick forward with the right. Continue explosively alternating kicks, never on more than one leg at a time.

* **Modification:** Lose the explosive movement and simply alternate kicks.

High Lows

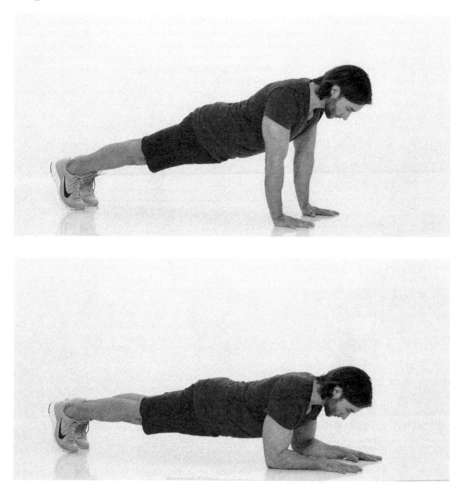

Assume a push-up position with wrists directly below the shoulders. Slowly lower the left forearm to the floor, elbow directly below the shoulder, and then the right. Return, one hand at a time, to the top of a push-up position. Continue lowering and raising.

Plié Jumps

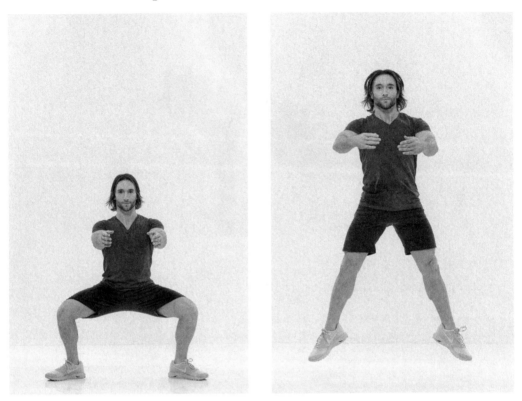

Stand with feet wider than shoulder-width apart, toes turned out wide. Keep your torso upright and core tight as you lower your hips down to at least knee level. Pause momentarily and explosively jump up, keeping your legs and feet wide to land in the starting position. Keep repeating.

* **Modification:** Lower and raise from starting position without jumping.

Squat Push-ups

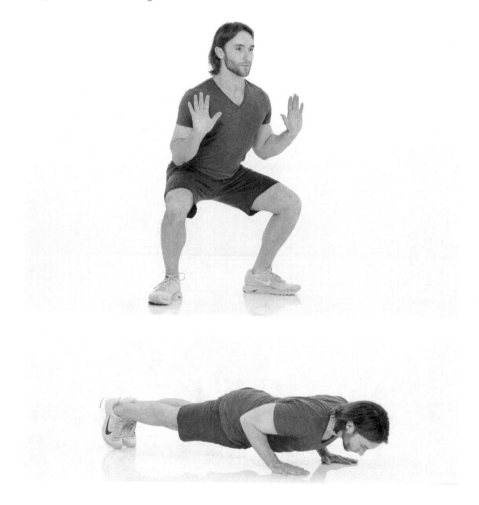

Start in a low squat. Drop the hands to the floor directly under your shoulders as you simultaneously kick your feet back to land in the top of a push-up position. Perform a push-up. At the top of the movement, jump the feet back to start and raise your chest up to pause momentarily in a low squat. Keep knees behind toes.

* **Modification:** Step the feet back and forward. Perform the push-up from your knees.

Deep Mountain Climbers

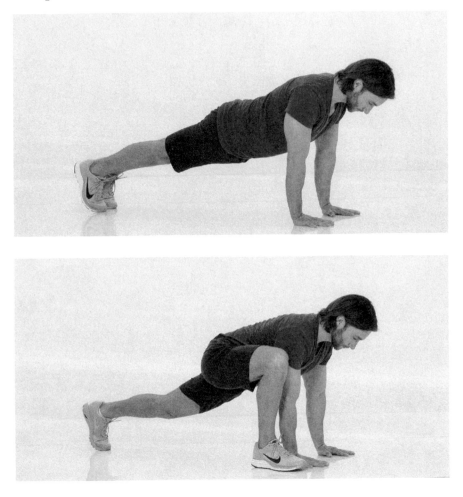

Start at the top of a push-up position. Step your right foot as close to the outside of your right hand as possible. Brace your core and explosively switch positions of your legs to land the right foot back and the left foot as close to the outside of the left hand as possible. Continue alternating.

* **Modification:** Step the feet, one at a time; don't explosively jump them.

Long-Jump Sprints

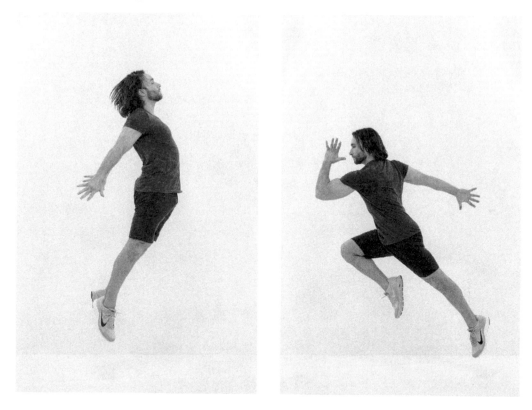

Stand with feet about hip-width apart. Pick a point on the floor in front of you and commit to jumping past it. Now brace your core as you lower down to a jump preparation position. Pause briefly at the bottom of the movement and explosively jump up and as far forward as you can. Land softly and sprint back to the starting position as fast as you can. Continue repeating the jump/run pattern.

* **Modification:** Take shorter jumps.

Table Saws

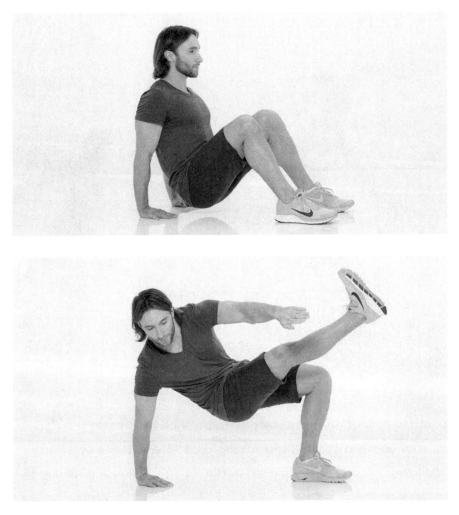

Sit on the floor with your knees bent and feet flat. Place your hands on the floor behind you, wrists under shoulders and fingers pointing toward your butt. Brace your core. Now press your hips straight up while simultaneously kicking the right foot up. At the same time, twist your torso to the right as you bring your left fingertips over the top of your toes. Imagine that you are trying to saw off your pinky toe with your pinky finger. Return to start and immediately repeat the movement on the opposite side. Continue alternating.

Laterals

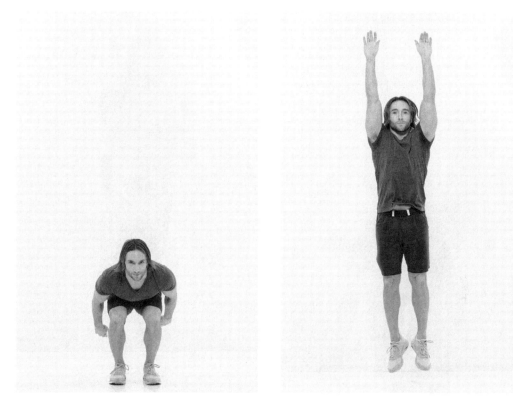

Start with your feet together and core tight. Press your hips back to lower your body and then explosively jump up and over as far as you can to the right, reaching fingertips to the sky. Land softly and lower your body, sweeping the ground with your fingertips. Immediately jump back to the starting position. That's 1 rep. Keep repeating.

* **Modification:** Take smaller jumps.

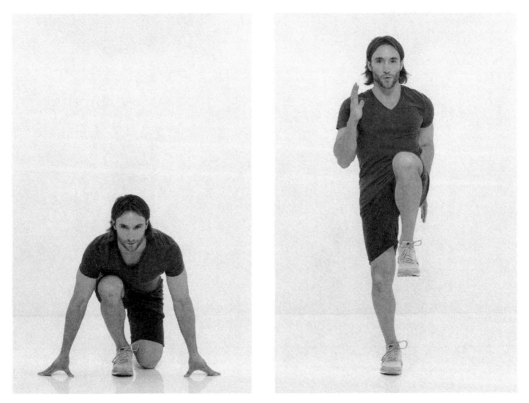

Sprint in place as fast as you can, pumping your arms and raising your knees to at least hip level.

* **Modification:** Slow down.

FiRE POWER

This is a fast and furious workout that cranks up the heat to leave you dripping in sweat.

Exercise	Time Duration

- Perform all moves back-to-back. Rest if/when you need to, but work up to doing all six exercises with no rest between moves.
- After you've completed all six moves, that's the end of Round 1.
- Rest 30 seconds and repeat twice more in this same format for three total rounds.
- Do not stop the timer.

Exercise	Time Duration	
Stickups	**30 seconds (Weeks 1–3)** 60 seconds (Weeks 4–6)	
Laterals	**30 seconds (Weeks 1–3)** 60 seconds (Weeks 4–6)	
Low Squat Sprints	**30 seconds (Weeks 1–3)** 60 seconds (Weeks 4–6)	HEAT 1
High Lows	**30 seconds (Weeks 1–3)** 60 seconds (Weeks 4–6)	
Low Plank Knees	**30 seconds (Weeks 1–3)** 60 seconds (Weeks 4–6)	
Power Kicks	**30 seconds (Weeks 1–3)** 60 seconds (Weeks 4–6)	

- Rest 30 seconds.
- Move on to Heat 2.
- Perform all moves below back-to-back. Rest if/when you need to.
- You're only doing 1 round of these moves below, so go hard!
- Work up to doing all the exercises with no rest between moves.
- Do not stop the timer.

Exercise	Time Duration
Standing Mountain Climbers	60 seconds
Pencil Squats	60 seconds
Power Thrusts	60 seconds
Muay Thais 30 seconds on each side, nonstop	60 seconds
Planker Taps 1 3-Point Planker/1 Tap-up	60 seconds
High Knee Jump Rope	60 seconds
Ladder Spiders 1 Ladder Climber/1 Spider Push-up	60 seconds
Box Jumps	60 seconds
High Plank Punches	60 seconds
Knees and Toes	60 seconds

• Complete only 1 round of the moves above.
• Rest 1 minute. Do your Cool Down.

HEAT 2

Stickups

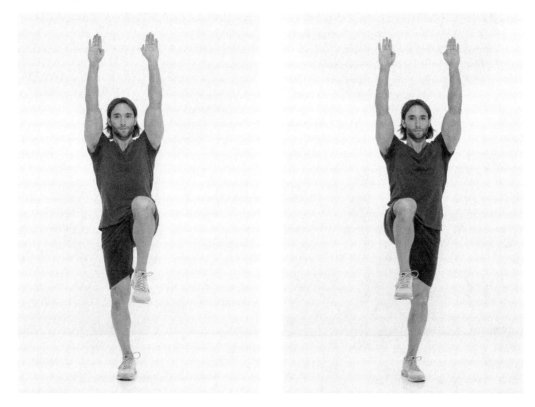

Stand tall with your feet hip-width apart and raise your fingertips to the sky. Spring in place, raising knees to at least hip height. Continue to alternate back and forth. Both knees = 1 rep.

Laterals

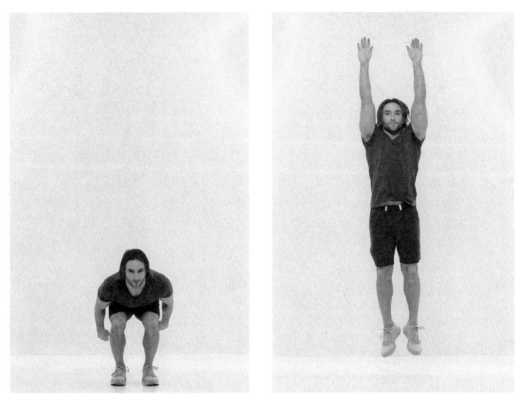

Start with your feet together and core tight. Press your hips back to lower your body and then explosively jump up and over as far as you can to the right, reaching fingertips to the sky. Land softly and lower your body, sweeping the ground with your fingertips. Immediately jump back to the starting position. That's 1 rep. Keep repeating.

* **Modification:** Take smaller jumps.

Low Squat Sprints

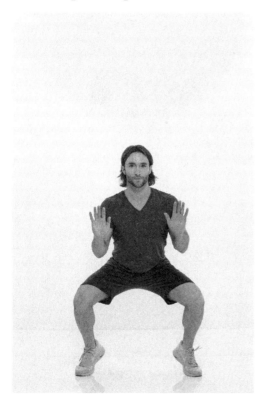

Start in a low squat with hips pressed back to at least knee level. Keep your chest up and chin parallel to the floor with your hands raised to chest level (as if you were going to stop someone from running into you). Raise up to the balls of your feet and sprint in place as fast as you can while alternately pumping the hands forward.

High Lows

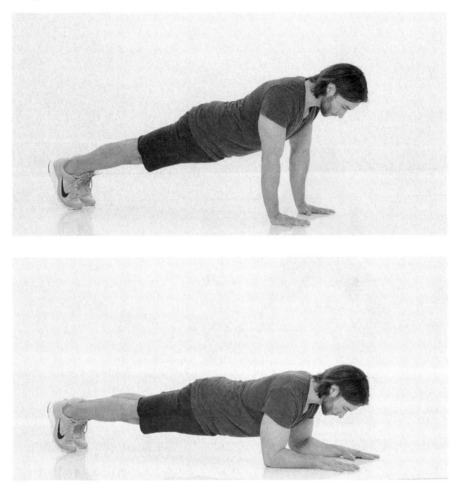

Assume a push-up position with wrists directly below the shoulders. Slowly lower the left forearm to the floor, elbow directly below the shoulder, and then the right. Return, one hand at a time, to the top of a push-up position. Continue lowering and raising.

Low Plank Knees

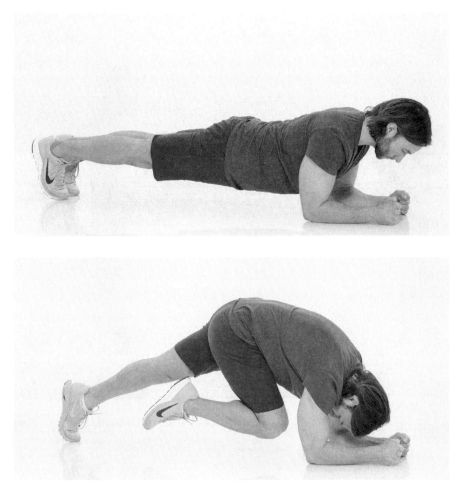

Assume a low plank position, forearms on the floor with elbows directly below shoulders. Pike your hips and drive your right knee toward your face and return to start. Repeat the motion on the opposite side. Continue alternating.

Power Kicks

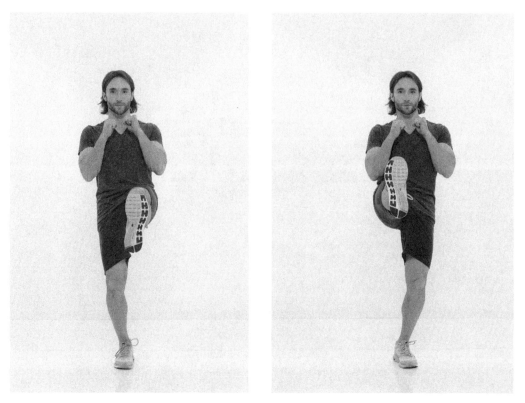

Stand with your feet slightly more than hip-width apart. Kick forward with your right foot up to at least hip level, extending through the heel. Explosively switch feet, lowering the right foot as you kick forward with the left. Continue alternating kicks, never on more than one leg at a time.

Standing Mountain Climbers

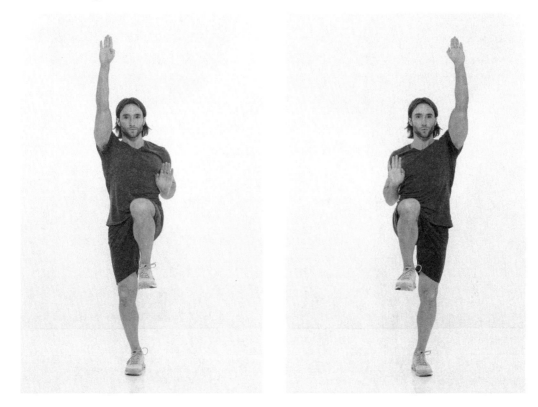

Stand with feet hip-width apart and hands in front of shoulders, palms facing forward. Brace your core and pull your shoulder blades down your back. Shoot your right fingertips to the sky as you raise your left knee up to hip height. Explosively switch sides, shooting the left fingertips to the sky as you raise your right knee to hip height. Continue alternating.

* **Modification:** Lose the explosive switch and simply alternate knee lifts while reaching the arms overhead.

Pencil Squats

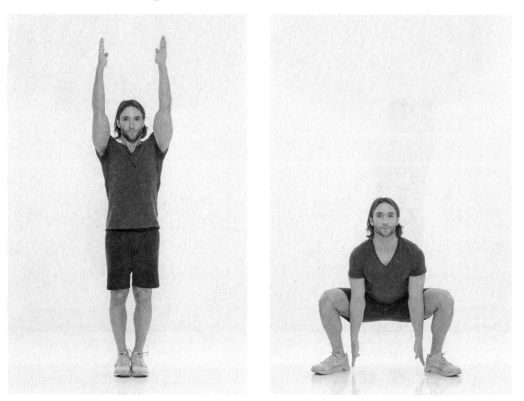

Stand with your feet together, arms raised overhead at shoulder width. Hop the feet apart to drop down into a low squat and touch the floor just behind your ankles. Explosively return to the starting position. Repeat.

* **Modification:** Lose the hops. Step out to the right, lower into a squat, and back to start. Arm movements are the same.

Power Thrusts

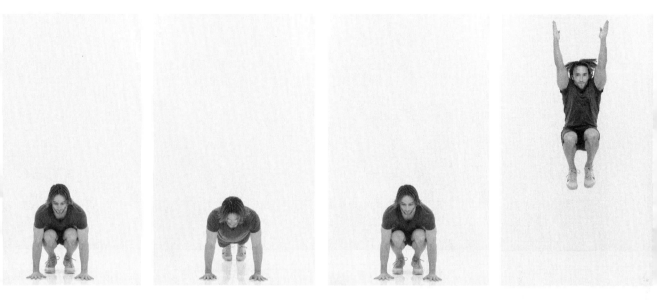

Stand with feet wider than hip-width apart. Squat down and place your hands on the floor, wrists positioned under your shoulders. Kick your feet back so that you're at the top of a push-up position. Immediately return them to the squat position. Explosively jump up off the floor, shooting your fingertips to the sky and driving your knees high up toward your chest. Land softly and quietly on the mid-foot, rolling back to the heels. Immediately push the hips back to absorb the impact of the landing. Repeat.

* **Modification:** Don't kick the feet back. Step back and then forward, one foot at a time. At the top of the movement, lose the jump and bring one knee at a time up to hip height with arms raised overhead.

Muay Thais

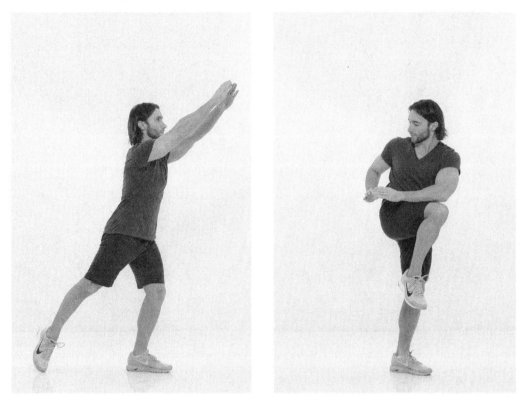

Stand with feet hip-width apart. Brace your core and extend your right leg out to the side, pointing your foot and resting the tip of your big toe on the floor. Reach your hands toward the corner of the ceiling in the opposite direction to form a straight line from fingertips to toes. Contract your core as you raise your right leg in to hip level. At the same time, bend your elbows and lower your arms until your left elbow meets your right thigh. Return to start. It may help to imagine that you're picking a coconut and then smashing it on the outside of your thigh. Continue repeating the movement on one side. Then switch sides and repeat.

Planker Taps

This is a combo move consisting of 1 3-Point Planker and 1 Tap-up.

3-POINT PLANKERS

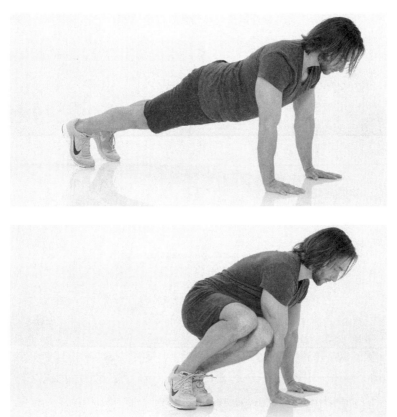

Assume a push-up position. Keep the hands flat on the floor and jump the feet as close as you can to the outside of the right hand. Return to start. Jump the feet as close as you can to the outside of the left hand. Return to start. Now jump the feet between the hands. Return to start. That's 1 rep. Continue repeating the move.

* **Modification:** Step the feet, one at a time, toward the hands and back, one at a time, to start.

TAP-UPS

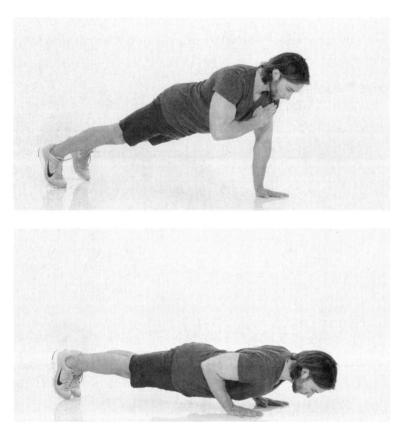

Assume a push-up position. Tap the left shoulder with right finger-tips and return the hand to the floor. Tap the right shoulder with the left fingertips and return the hand to the floor. Perform a push-up. Repeat.

High Knee Jump Rope

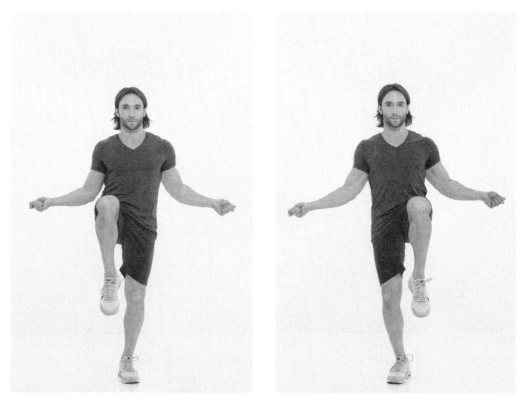

While swinging an imaginary jump rope, raise one knee up as high as you can, then repeat on the other side. Pretend the rope is real and sync the rope hitting the floor with your skips. Continue alternating.

Ladder Spiders

This is a combo move consisting of 1 Ladder Climber and 3 Spiders.

LADDER CLIMBERS

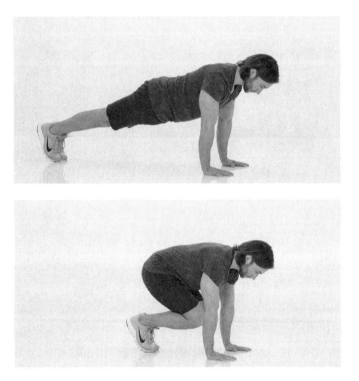

Assume a push-up position. Imagine that your body is above a ladder with your hands on the outsides of it and your feet at the bottom. Keep your hands flat on the floor, brace your core, and jump the feet forward about 1 foot, as if you were jumping them into the first box of the ladder. Return to start. Jump the feet forward about 2 feet, as if into the second box of the ladder. Return to start. Now jump the feet close to the hands, as if into the third box of the ladder. Jump the feet back to start. Continue repeating.

* **Modification:** Step the feet forward and then back, one foot at a time.

SPIDERS

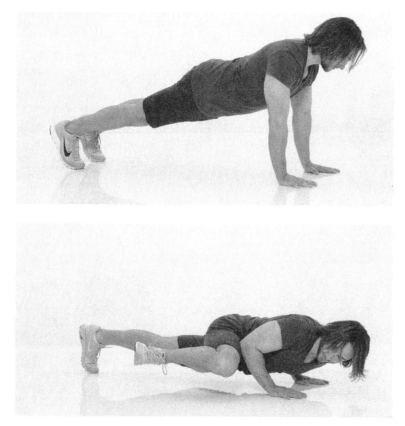

Assume a push-up position with wrists directly under the shoulders. Bend the elbows straight back to lower the chest to 1 inch above the floor. As you lower, bring the right knee in toward the right elbow. Press back up to start. Repeat the motion with the left knee. That's 1 rep.

* **Modification:** Perform the move with your knees on the floor. To further modify, perform regular push-ups.

Box Jumps

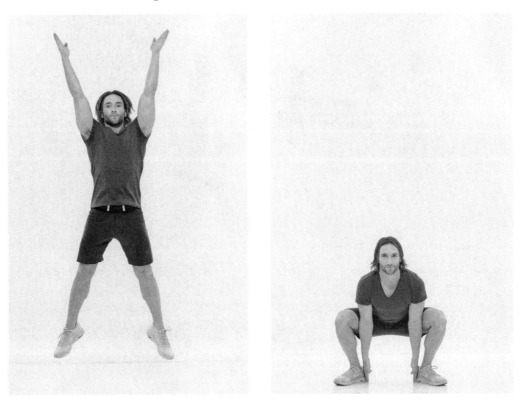

Imagine a large square drawn on the floor. You're standing on the back right corner of it. Press your hips back to lower into a squat. Pause briefly at the bottom of the movement and explosively jump forward into the front right corner of the "square." Land softly and press your hips back into a low squat. Repeat the movement, this time jumping to the left to land on the front left corner of the "square." Repeat the movement, this time jumping backward to the back left corner of the "square." Now jump right to return to the starting point. That's 1 rep. Continue the pattern.

* **Modification:** Take smaller jumps.

High Plank Punches

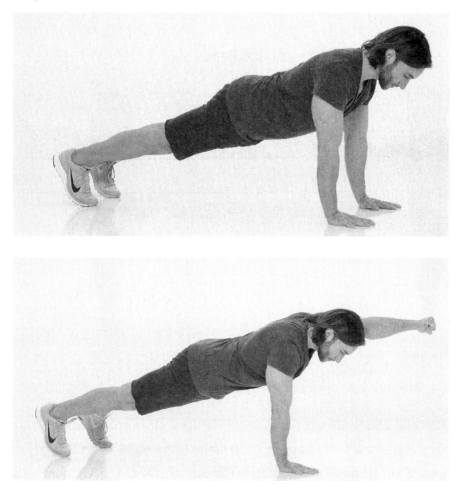

Assume a plank position with wrists directly under shoulders. Punch forward with the left fist at shoulder level. Place hand back on floor. Repeat with the right fist.

Knees and Toes

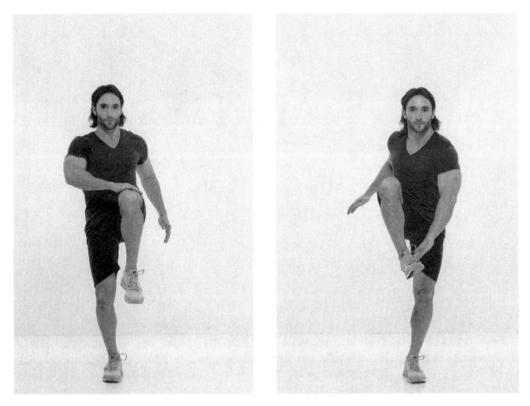

Run one round of high knees (left knee, then right knee up to at least hip level), touching the left knee with right hand and right knee with left hand. Immediately repeat, this time driving the knees higher to tap the left toes with right fingers and right toes with left fingers. Keep cycling through the movements, tapping knee, knee, toes, toes.

Cool Down

After each of these workouts, it's important to gradually cool the body down while lengthening out the muscles you just worked. Skip your post-workout stretches and you may find yourself with all sorts of pain and trouble. So bang out this simple cooldown routine, holding each stretch for five breaths.

All the moves below should be performed back-to-back, with a sense of flow. Make sure to keep the knees soft, never fully locked; and always keep the body nice and easy, without any tightness or tension.

Arm Sweep

Inhale as you sweep your arms up overhead, joining the palms together at the top. Exhale and you draw your hands down to the center of your chest.

* Repeat 3 times.

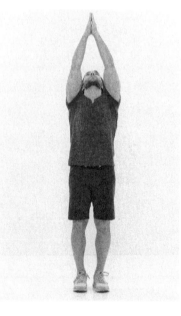

Side Bend

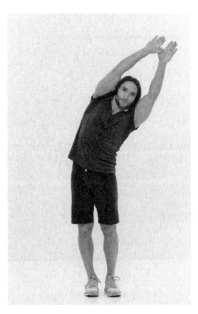

Perform the arm sweep above. This time, at the top of the movement, hook the thumbs together and extend the fingertips over to the left. You should feel the right side of the body lengthen out. Hold for 3 breaths. Return to center on an inhale. Exhale as you take it over to the other side. Hold for 3 breaths. Return to center.

Tri Pry

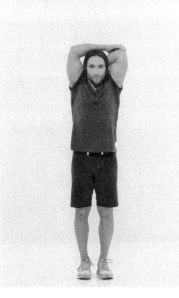

With arms extended overhead, drop the left forearm behind the head. Gently take hold of the left arm just above the elbow on the triceps, pressing gently to lengthen. Hold for 5 breaths. Straighten the arm back out. Repeat with the right arm.

Forward Bend

Perform the arm sweep above. This time, allow the hands to continue to move past the chest as you bend forward at the hips to touch the floor, bending the knees as necessary. Let your neck relax and head hang heavy. Hold for 5 breaths.

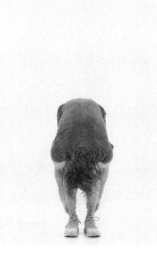

Standing Flat Back

Inhale as you look forward and lengthen out your torso to come up to a flat back. There should be a 90-degree angle from your heels to hips to head. Your fingertips can be on the ground, your shins, or your thighs—whichever is most comfortable. Hold for 5 breaths.

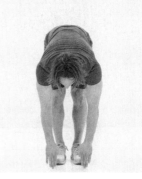

Hip Flex

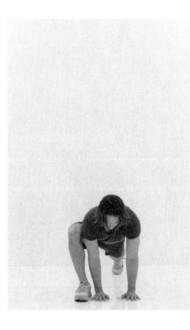

Inhale as you bend your knees; place your palms flat on the ground and step your left foot back into a deep lunge. Be sure to keep the right knee directly over the right ankle. Keep the hands flat on the floor, knuckles in line with the arch of the foot. Open the chest and pull the shoulders down the back. You should feel a nice stretch in the hip. Hold for 5 breaths. Now inhale as you step the left foot forward to meet the right. Then step the right foot back into a deep lunge. Same positioning as on the other side. Hold for 5 breaths. Then step the right foot forward to meet the left.

Straddle

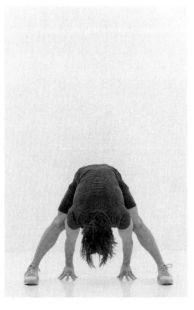

From here, step the right foot out to the right so that your legs are in a wide straddle. Straighten out the legs and bend at the hips to let your torso hang heavy. Fingertips can be on the floor. If the backs of your legs feel really tight, you can place the hands on the thighs. Hold for 5 breaths.

Side Straddle

From here, take the hands over to the outside of the left foot. Be sure to lead with the chest, not the head, keeping the neck in line with the spine. If this is uncomfortable, you can place the hands on the shin or thigh. Hold for 5 breaths and inhale as you take it over to the right. Hold for another 5 breaths. Inhale as you come to center. Bend the knees and slowly heel-toe the feet together.

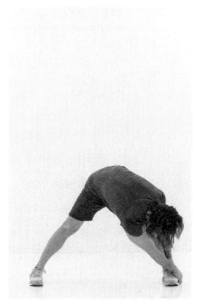

Rise and Shine

With knees soft, tuck the chin to the chest and roll up slowly one vertebra at a time, letting the head be the last thing to come up. As your head comes up, sweep the arms up overhead, joining the palms together, looking up at your hands. Close your eyes as you exhale and draw the palms to the center of your chest. With your eyes closed, open the chest wide and pull the shoulders down your back. Take 3 deep breaths here. Exhale your third breath as you open your eyes. Now go have a beautiful day!

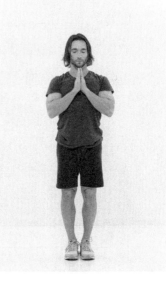

Recovery Yoga

When you're working out regularly, and just walking around living your daily life, your muscles get tight. Consistently tight muscles are a one-way ticket to a place I like to call InjuryTown. You don't want to live there. You don't even want to visit.

To make matters worse, there's a good chance you spend a large portion of your day sitting at a desk in front of a computer. If that's the case and you're not stretching regularly, you are *really* setting yourself up for an injury or at the very least some nagging lower back pain.

Yoga is the one of the best ways to maintain mobility and flexibility for life. This beginner's routine is a crucial part of the program—just as important for achieving a fit body as those intense intervals—so please, never skip this day!

Below, you'll find four simple sequences. They can be mixed and matched depending on what your time allows. Pair two or three of them together for a successful stretch that will target your entire body and allow your muscles and joints to rest and recover, ready and primed for the rest of the week's workouts!

Whichever sequences you choose, make sure you finish with a well-earned round of Shavasana.

Shoulder Stretch Warm-Up (3 min.)

1. EASY SEATED POSE—
SUKHASANA

Begin in a super-comfortable, cross-legged seated position. If it's difficult to sit on the floor for any reason, prop your seat up with a cushion or a pillow.

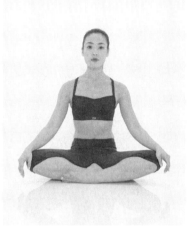

This is Wendy! She's an amazing athlete, dancer, Yogi, and friend. She's also on the cover of the book!

2. PRAYER HANDS—
ANJALI OR NAMASTE MUDRA

Put your hands in prayer at your chest. Take a sec to give thanks. You've made it to Wednesday!

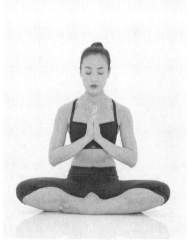

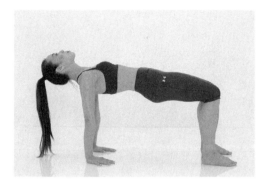

3. TABLE TOP POSE— PURVOTTANASANA (VARIATION)

Place feet flat on the floor, hip distance apart. Place the hands on the floor just behind the hips with the fingers facing forward. Lift the hips up until the body is flat from the shoulders to the knees. Press the tailbone toward the ceiling to focus the stretch on both the front of the hips and the shoulders. Come back down to the seated position.

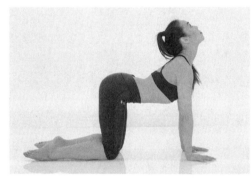

4. CAT AND COW STRETCH

From a seated position, roll forward and come to your hands and knees. Move with the breath. Inhale, drop the chest and belly to arch the back and look up. Exhale, round the back, and try to look toward the navel. Continue with a few breaths and feel free to introduce some circular movements to the spine as long as it feels awesome.

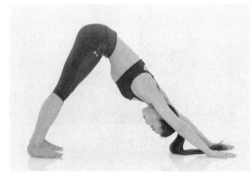

5. DOWNWARD FACING DOG— ADHO MUKHA SVANASANA

While on the hands and knees, make sure the shoulders are over the wrists and the hips over the knees to ensure proper alignment. Tuck the toes and lift the hips while also pressing them backward. In the beginning, keep the knees bent like a cat ready to pounce, to allow the back to straighten and alleviate the weight in the wrists. Over time, the knees will straighten to bring even more of a stretch into the hamstrings and calves. Press the heels toward the floor and create space between the shoulders and the ears. From someone else's perspective, you will look like an inverted V in this shape. From your perspective you'll just look like a badass.

6. FORWARD FOLD—UTTANASANA

From Downward Facing Dog, walk the feet forward to meet the hands. It's okay to bend the knees along the way. Bring the feet hip distance apart and grab opposite elbows to allow the upper spine to release. Soften the neck and tuck the chin slightly to lengthen the all-too-often-crunched cervical spine. Try straightening the legs to release the hamstrings and the lower back.

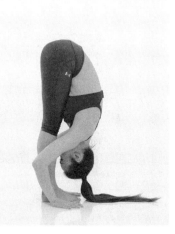

7. MOUNTAIN POSE— TADASANA (SAMASTHITI)

Stand up. Place the feet firmly underneath you. Allow the arms to drop to the sides of the body. Be proud and let it show.

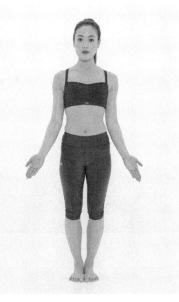

Slow Sun Salutation (4 min.)

This is your recovery day, so take it easy. Spend a little time in the poses, let them stretch you out and feel good. There's no "winning" on this one. You're welcome to do one simple Slow Sun Salutation, or several. It depends on what time and your body allow.

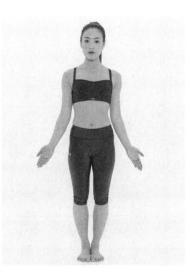

1. MOUNTAIN POSE— TADASANA (SAMASTHITI)

Start with arms at sides and good posture. Notice how you feel in your body as you stand here, with the feet firmly planted, chest open, and arms at the sides. Take a few deep breaths and see how the breath changes the shape of the muscles and your frame.

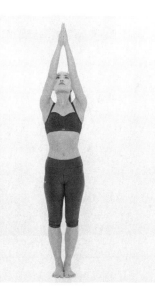

2. ARMS UP—URDHVA HASTASANA

Reach the arms above the head and keep the shoulders moving down away from the ears. Lift the lower belly in and up to prevent collapsing into the lower back.

3. FORWARD FOLD—UTTANASANA

Bend forward at the hips and place the hands on the floor. Bend the knees if necessary.

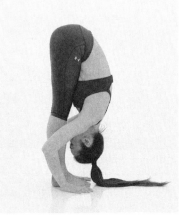

4. FLAT BACK POSITION— ARDHA UTTANASANA

Inhale, and lengthen the spine so that it is straight. At this point, the knees may bend slightly, and the hands may come to the shins. Keep the back of the neck long.

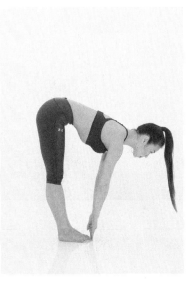

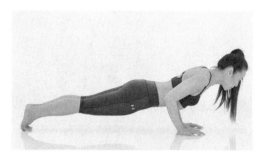

5. FOUR-LEGGED STAFF POSE— CHATURANGA DANDASANA

Place the hands firmly on the floor underneath the shoulders and walk the feet back into a plank position with the body nice and straight. Exhale, and lower into a low push-up position, but make sure the elbows are by the sides, and the body is in a flat, plank-like shape. Make sure the core is engaged throughout this pose.

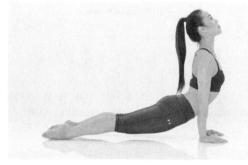

6. UPWARD FACING DOG— URDHVA MUKHA SVANASANA

From Four-Legged Staff (low push-up), straighten the arms and lift the chest. Come into a backbend shape and flip the feet so the toes point directly behind you. Engage the quadriceps and lift the knees off the floor to protect the lower back. Keep the back of the neck long as you allow the entire front side of the body to stretch.

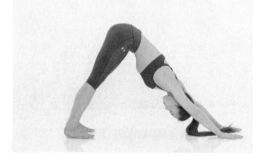

7. DOWNWARD FACING DOG— ADHO MUKHA SVANASANA

Carefully turn the feet over and lift the hips up and back into Downward Facing Dog. As you go, keep the core engaged to protect the lower back as you transition into this pose. Reach the heels toward the floor and feel free to bend the knees if the back is rounded. Imagine an upside-down V shape—this is what you're aiming to create with your body. Tuck the chin slightly to lengthen the back of the neck.

8. FLAT BACK POSITION— ARDHA UTTANASANA

From Downward Facing Dog, step the feet up between the hands and inhale into a Flat Back Position. Lengthen the spine, and bend the knees if needed.

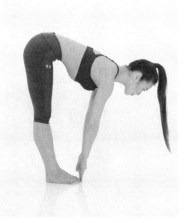

9. FORWARD FOLD—UTTANASANA

From the Flat Back Position, exhale and fold forward, tucking the chin and aiming the forehead to the shins. No worries if it doesn't get there. Place the goal in your mind and use the breath to embody as much of it as you can. What matters less is the outer shape. What matters more is the inner tenacity.

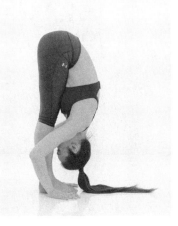

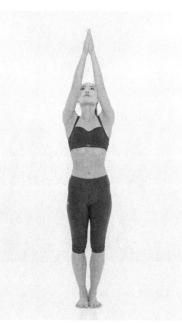

10. ARMS UP—URDHVA HASTASANA

Reach the arms up to the sky and lengthen and stretch the entire body. Reach for it. Go. Press the feet down and stay grounded as you do.

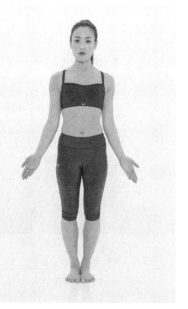

11. MOUNTAIN POSE— TADASANA (SAMASTHITI)

Back where we started, coming full circle. Find good posture and stand proudly.

Relax the Back (4 min.)

1. DOWNWARD FACING DOG— ADHO MUKHA SVANASANA

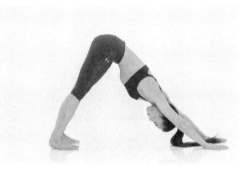

Place the hands shoulder-distance apart on the floor and the knees under the hips. Tuck the toes and lift the hips up and back as you work to straighten the spine, bending the knees if necessary. Reach the heels to the floor and tuck the chin. This posture helps to stretch the entire back side of the body.

2. LYING DOWN BIG TOE STRETCH— SUPTA PADANGHUSTHASANA

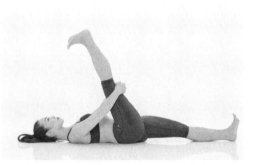

From Downward Facing Dog, come onto the hands and knees and then make your way onto your back. Lie down and extend the left leg onto the floor with the quads engaged and the toes pointing straight up. Hug the right knee into the chest and interlace the fingers behind the right thigh. Straighten the right leg, reaching the right heel toward the ceiling as you draw the leg toward the body, stretching out the hamstrings and the lower back. Keep the shoulders relaxed and on the floor. Relax the neck and the jaw. Find your happy place. Breathe. Switch sides.

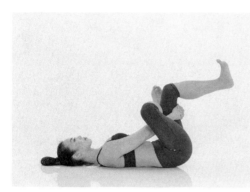

3. THREAD-THE-NEEDLE STRETCH

While lying on the back, hug the knees into the chest. Place the right ankle on the left knee, allowing the right knee to open to the right side. Reach the right hand through the legs and interlace both sets of fingers behind the left thigh as you draw the left knee and right shin toward the chest. Keep the shoulders on the floor. Feel a stretch in your right outer hip? Say hello to your piriformis. Your athletic performance will thank you for doing this stretch. Breathe into the stretch to allow it to open. Switch sides.

Release the Hips (4 min.)

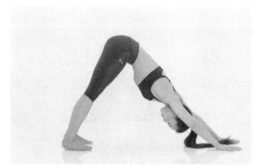

1. DOWNWARD FACING DOG— ADHO MUKHA SVANASANA

Place the hands shoulder-distance apart on the floor and the knees under the hips. By now, you know what to do. See if each time you come into Downward Facing Dog, the quintessential yoga pose, you can find more muscles to release and soften, aiming for a feeling of ease and calm in the shape.

2. PIGEON STRETCH—
RAJA KAPOTASANA (VARIATION)

Bring the left knee just behind the left wrist and lower the hips to the floor, with the right leg stretched behind you. To dial the stretch up a notch, make the left shin parallel with the front of your yoga mat. To ease off on the stretch, bring the left ankle more under the left hip. In any case, make sure there is no pain or pressure in the left knee. Square the hips off to the front of the mat and settle the torso down, either resting on the elbows or stretching the arms out in front of you on the floor. Breathe into the stretch in the hips. Switch sides. Finish both sides by coming back to Downward Facing Dog.

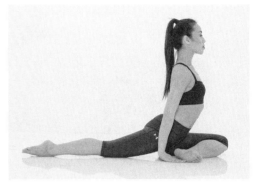

3. BOUND ANGLE POSE—
BADDHA KONASANA

From Downward Facing Dog, bring the knees to the floor and come to a comfortable seated position. Place the feet flat on the floor together and bring them close to your seat. Allow the knees to fall apart as the bottoms of the feet press together. Grab the feet and fold forward over the legs. If the knees are high off the floor, it is wise to put pillows or blankets under them to allow the hips to open more easily. It's okay to round the back in this pose; however, try to keep the shoulders away from the ears and the upper back and neck soft.

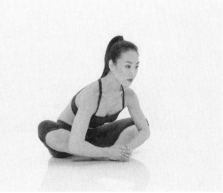

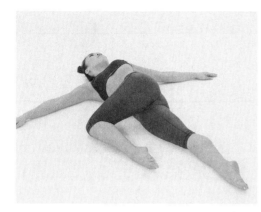

4. SUPINE SPINAL TWIST— JATHARA PARIVRTTASANA

From Bound Angle Pose, lift the knees up using both hands and roll down onto the back, hugging the knees into the chest. You can remain here for a few breaths, doing some circles with the knees to relax the lower back and upper body. Hug the left knee to the chest and extend the right leg out onto the floor. Twist the torso by dropping the left knee to the right side with the right hand on the knee. Reach the left arm out behind you and gaze over the left shoulder. Imagine the twist originating at the top of the head all the way to the right heel. Breathe here for a few moments. Switch sides. Finish by hugging the knees into the chest.

Shavasana

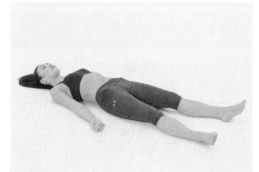

Best. Yoga. Pose. Ever. This is the way yoga practitioners always finish their practice. It allows the benefits of the practice to be absorbed by all levels of the body. Take your time in this pose, and for goodness' sake, don't skip it! You've earned it and you deserve a moment's peace.

Lie on the floor on your back and extend your body on the floor in the shape of the classic Vetruvian Man (à la Michelangelo). Bring the feet wider than hip-distance apart and allow the hands to rest, palms up, at the sides.

Use the breath and the awareness to go through the entire body, muscle by muscle, bone by bone, organ by organ, to make sure that every piece of tissue is completely relaxed. Then relax your brain. Rather than focusing on the thoughts, simply focus on the breath and let go.

Remain here for as long as you like.

Bonus! 5-Minute Quick Fires

This isn't part of the outlined plan, but I want to give you something extra and make 100 percent sure that you never miss a workout. (Not that you would do that anyway, right? Come on! It's only 6 short weeks!) These little gems take only 5 minutes and will leave you totally spent. You can do just one or repeat or stack a few of them for a longer session as your time allows.

- Choose any of the three workouts below.
- Perform all 5 moves back-to-back. No rest.
- Repeat or stack multiple workouts for a longer session. If doing so, rest 30 seconds between rounds.

Exercise	Time Duration
Knees and Toes	60 seconds
Tuck Jumps	60 seconds
Tap-ups	60 seconds
3-Point Plankers	60 seconds
High Knee Jump Rope	60 seconds

WORKOUT 1

Exercise	Time Duration
Oblique High Knees	60 seconds
Power Thrusts	60 seconds
Spiders	60 seconds
Laterals	60 seconds
Deep Mountain Climbers	60 seconds

WORKOUT 2

Exercise	Time Duration
Stickups	60 seconds
Long-Jump Sprints	60 seconds
Ladder Climbers	60 seconds
Pencil Squats	60 seconds
High Plank Punches	60 seconds

WORKOUT 3

REST. iT WORKS.

HERE'S SOMETHING THAT MAY COME AS A surprise: When you're working out, you're not actually *building* muscle—you're tearing it down. Think about it like building a house. The workout is the demolition crew. The rest period is the builder. It's during the periods of rest that your body actually builds muscle, repairing the damaged tissue into a longer, leaner, stronger you. Wanna be all toned and sexy? You have to properly rest.

Working out every day not only causes burnout, it can also lead to overtraining. This is an actual condition where you stop making progress and can even start to lose strength and conditioning.

You'll notice the seventh day on your workout calendar says Pure Rest. You've been working your butt off. So enjoy the break. And really, these workouts don't take that long so it's not like this suddenly gives you more hours in the day to do a bunch of stuff that you've been missing out on. That's kind of the point. You crush these short workouts and still have time to live a full, fun life! This day is more about letting your body fully recover.

Spend some time today reflecting on the previous week's successes and commit to kicking up your intensity a notch in the coming week. Whatever you do, enjoy yourself fully! Your body will thank you for it, and be stronger come Monday.

SHOWER. RiNSE. REPEAT.

WHAT TO DO ONCE YOU'VE CRUSHED THE six weeks? First, jump up and down (you can do this significantly higher and longer than before—pretty cool, right?), pat yourself on the back, and take a moment to bask in the glory of finishing this challenge. You're part of our tribe now. A merry band of misfits, rock stars, and general badasses who've taken control of their bodies and lives. You're fit; you're fierce; you're . . . well . . . you're you!

Second, don't forget to take your third set of photos and measurements!

Third, I'd recommend taking a week of *active recovery* to reflect on your goals. Are you where you want to be? Do you want to change up your routine in any way? Assess and proceed accordingly. *Active recovery* means setting aside hard workouts in favor of lighter fare, like long bike rides or hikes, some pickup sports, etc. It's not a week of sitting on your butt and regressing. After this six-week program you'll have ignited a sense of momentum and physical conditioning that's nearly impossible to abandon. So take pride in your new physique and strength, and keep on moving!

Always remember Newton's first law of motion: A body at rest will remain at rest and a body in motion will remain in motion. (I condensed the full quote for brevity, but you get the point.)

After that active rest week, you can most certainly jump right back into another 6-Week Challenge. Remember, you're going for time, not reps—so you'll always be pushed to your max and forced to grow. Keep your first Fit Test results handy and measure them up against the results in your second 6-Week Challenge. As you get stronger, you'll be able to do more reps in the allotted time and it will feel truly amazing to see yourself progress. Nothing wrong with a little one-on-one competition!

Whatever you choose, I want to say *Congrats!* In my mind right now, I'm giving you a massive high-five and telling all my friends and family about how you just crushed this challenge and earned your best body. I hope you're doing the same.

30-SECOND BODY 6-Week Workout Calendar

	Monday	Tuesday	Wednesday	Thursday	Friday	Saturday	Sunday
Week 1	Photos and Measurements 1 Fit Test 1	Cardio Blaze	Airborne	Recovery Yoga	Fire Power	Airborne	Pure Rest
Week 2	Cardio Blaze	Fire Power	Airborne	Recovery Yoga	Cardio Blaze	Fire Power	Pure Rest
Week 3	Fit Test 2	Airborne	Fire Power	Recovery Yoga	Cardio Blaze	Airborne	Photos and Measurements 2 —— Pure Rest

	Monday	Tuesday	Wednesday	Thursday	Friday	Saturday	Sunday
Week 4	Cardio Blaze	Airborne	Fire Power	Recovery Yoga	Fire Power	Cardio Blaze	Pure Rest
Week 5	Airborne	Cardio Blaze	Fire Power	Recovery Yoga	Cardio Blaze	Airborne	Pure Rest
Week 6	Fire Power	Airborne	Cardio Blaze	Recovery Yoga	Airborne	Fit Test 3	Photos and Measurements 3 — Pure Rest

* Available as a printout at www.the30secondbody.com.

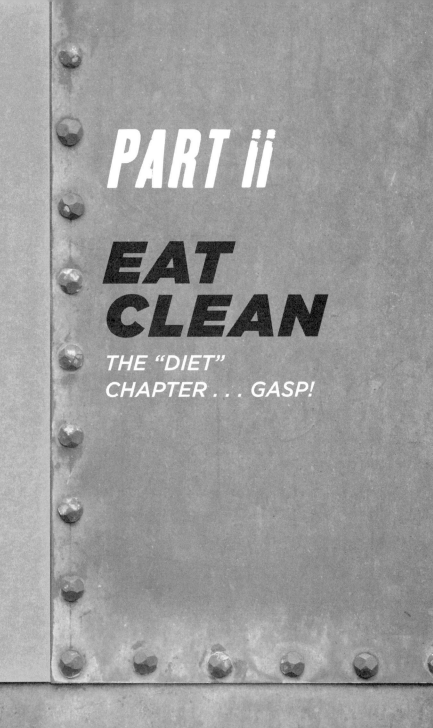

PART ii

EAT CLEAN

*THE "DIET"
CHAPTER . . . GASP!*

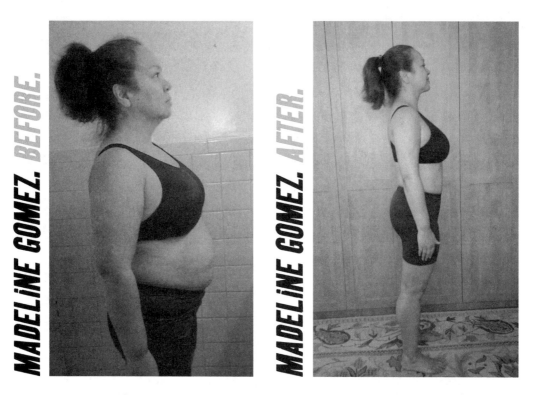

MADELINE GOMEZ. BEFORE.

MADELINE GOMEZ. AFTER.

"This came at a time when I really needed to get moving and start working out again. Real talk? Depression is a bitch. I had stopped working out and I had lost my motivation to do so. I needed something different to shake me out of my funk and the usual 'lift up, put down' routine was not it. So I jumped at the chance to challenge myself and try Adam's workout. It was one of the best decisions I could have ever made. I looked forward to each and every workout each week. It was challenging, invigorating, and boy-oh-boy what a sweat fest of a workout. It is a challenge, but the feeling you get after you are done is priceless. His guidance on how to eat eliminates confusion and keeps it simple without keeping you hungry. And even though his workouts seriously kick your butt, at the end of the day, you'll smile and feel the need to thank him."

THiS WON'T HURT A BiT

TAKE A DEEP BREATH. NOW EXHALE.

I promise that this is going to be pretty painless. The truth is that eating right to lose weight isn't nearly as difficult or complicated as you've been led to believe. But any trip to the bookstore or time spent trolling fitness blogs will leave your head spinning. There's simply too much information out there. A lot of it's conflicting, much of it is confusing, and all of it combined is overwhelming.

Here's the thing: A lot of the programs and "fad diets" out there will work to help you lose some weight in the short term. But that's the catch. It's all in the *short term*. A fad, by definition, is meant to pass. And as with the boy bands of the nineties, you're going to get sick of whatever fad you've been sold. And once you tire of it, if it's weight you've lost, I can guarantee that it's weight you'll find again.

I may have started this book with the fitness program, but here's a simple fact: No matter how hard you work out, you can't out-train a bad diet. A lean body is built on smart eating habits and great food. Any other approach is like building a house on a cardboard foundation. Sooner or later, it's going to crumble.

The "diet" in *The 30-Second Body* isn't a diet at all. It's about eating real food five times a day and loving it. Rather than overwhelming you with confusing equations or complex nutritional patterns, we're going to put our focus on a few digestible (pun intended) and actionable steps that you can take to start losing weight this week. My big-picture goal is for you to take these *steps,* add a little *thought,* and be *self-sufficient.* There's no counting calories or measuring out protein grams on a scale (if you'd even do that sort of thing) or drinking some weird witch's potion to lose weight.

I'm asking you to listen to your body. That may sound a little esoteric and soft, but it's important that you get in tune with yourself. There's a ridiculously simple way to "measure" your food portions so that you get the right amount without ever counting calories. At first, some folks are a little put off by how easy it seems, but trust me here. As you progress over the course of the upcoming weeks, ask yourself, "How do I feel?" "How is this working for me?" If the answer to both of those questions is "Great!" then stay the course. If you find that you're really, really hungry, losing *too* much weight (don't roll your eyes and laugh, I hear this sometimes), or what I'm suggesting is too much food for you to consume, then adjust accordingly. Basically, eat a little more or eat a little less. I'm not there to watch your every move. You're an awesome, responsible, intelligent human being. You got this!

And sure, you could guzzle some concoction that sounds like something I would have made in my grandma's kitchen as a child pretending to be a mad scientist, exclude any number of nutritious foods, like most diets du jour recommend, or shun carbs altogether. You *could* do that. And you'd likely lose some pounds. But there's a pretty good (I'd say nearly certain) chance that you'll gain it all back and then some. Trust me, there's an easier way to lose the weight and keep it off for life.

Now, I'd be a far richer man if I had a dollar for every time someone said to me, "Adam, I literally just want to be told what to do. Just give me a list of recipes."

I understand where you're coming from. There are days where I look at all that I have to do and get so overwhelmed I could scream. I am going to spell out exactly what you should do to succeed in your weight loss goals, but I don't want you to just mindlessly follow a meal plan. I want you to be self-sufficient. What happens when my recipes run out? You'll undoubtedly repeat some of them—they're delicious, after all—putting a few into regular rotation for a while, but eventually you're going to want something new. That's when it's easy to fall off the wagon. Don't put yourself in a position where you're back to looking for the next magic trick. When you understand *how* to eat, you're in control forever.

These principles won't overwhelm you, but will rather equip you to venture confidently into the often-confusing realm of eating well. You know as well as I do how frustrating it is; otherwise you wouldn't be holding this book. To use a tired metaphor, this is me teaching you how to fish rather than giving you a grilled sea bass. If you invest a little more effort than the average bear and follow the guidelines below, you'll be, well, happier, healthier, and hotter than the average bear. And to further enable your self-sufficiency, at the end of this chapter I'm going to give you a blueprint for what I call a *Clean Power Smoothie*. In just six easy steps you'll have more nutrition in you than most people get in a week.

So no more feeling confused and overwhelmed, okay? The simple info below is your easy-to-follow road map. Let's grab the wheel and go for a joyride!

12 SIMPLE KEYS TO MASTER YOUR "DIET"

#1 *Good Food Goes Bad*

If you want to lose weight and keep it off without making yourself miserable, you need to eat the *right* foods. And just what *are* the right foods? Simple: whole foods. No, not the store (though it is a lovely place). I'm talking about *food as close to its natural state as possible.* You know, food that goes bad quickly. Single-word foods that have been plucked from nature and slapped with a price sticker: say, avocadoes, broccoli, or sweet potatoes. They're the opposite of that processed stuff that's just *passing* for food. You know, those boxes with ingredient lists the length of the Nile. Like Rice-A-Roni, Frosted Flakes, or a box of mac and cheese. You've got some sitting in your pantry right now, don't you? That's okay. We'll take care of that later.

Write this phrase down and stick it on your fridge: *good foods go bad,* or, if you'd rather, *food as close to its natural state as possible.* Seriously, set this book down for one minute, grab a piece of paper and a pen, write one of those phrases down, and stick it on your refrigerator. While you're at it, type out another one in your phone. That phrase is going to be your filter for food choices from now on.

Okay, you did it, right? It wasn't a rhetorical exercise. Don't be that person who reads this book for inspiration, but never takes any action. The first few steps of any new adventure are always the hardest. Force yourself to take them.

If you're looking at this exercise and thinking, *Adam, this is lame,* good! It's not a trick. I want you to realize how simple it is to identify good food from bad.

Pantry Raid

What's the easiest way to avoid temptation? Remove it.

Go through your refrigerator, pantry, and cabinets and throw out all the items that don't align with that phrase above. Feeling shameful about wasting food? Don't. I'll dive into that later. For now, be ruthless. If it doesn't go bad and if it isn't as close to its natural state as possible, it goes in the trash. Once it's all gone, give your fridge, kitchen, and cabinets a thorough cleaning. As you're cleaning I want you to imagine that you're cleaning up your mind and your body, preparing it for all the fresh, nutrient-rich foods you're about to provide. Be proud of this choice you've made to live a healthy, active lifestyle. Then hit the grocery store and stock up on clean, lean food.

Now, don't bug out. I'm not so out-of-touch to demand that every single thing you put into your body be grown in your backyard or purchased from the farmer's market. If that's what you can swing, amazing (and please invite me over for dinner; I'll help cook and even do the dishes after!). If not, no worries. You can find whole foods at your local grocery store. You see, I'm not suggesting you cut out food that's sold in packages. That's both unrealistic and unnecessary. Ever get a bag of baby spinach? That's *food as close to its natural state as possible*. It fits the phrase "good foods go bad." It just happens to be in a package.

When it comes to buying packaged food containing more than a single ingredient, I'm a big fan of the "five-ingredient rule," which Michael Pollan wrote about in his book *Food Rules.* Five isn't a magic number per se, but when you choose foods with five ingredients or fewer, you are likely choosing unprocessed foods. Recipes with more than five ingredients aren't necessarily bad as long as each ingredient is as close to its natural state as possible—and if you're making food at home, that's always going to be better for you than something you buy in a store or restaurant.

On the other hand, if you're in the grocery store and you pick up a box of something with a list of ingredients that would require a PhD in chemical engineering to decipher, that's not cool. Remember, good food goes bad. Really think about that. If something is able to sit on a shelf in the grocery store or your pantry for months at a time, do you really want whatever's in there inside your body? I certainly don't.

When scrutinizing packages, keep in mind that ingredients on a food label are listed according to their weight. Those first few ingredients make up the majority of what's inside. It really puts things in perspective when several forms of sugar or unrecognizable "Frankengredients" are up top. Remember: *good foods go bad* and *food as close to its natural state as possible*. Is the food you're about to purchase as close to its natural state as possible, or is it some barely recognizable version of the real thing? Proceed accordingly.

A quick example? Sweet potatoes versus frozen sweet potato fries. A sweet potato is nothing more than a sweet potato. Cut it up, toss it with olive oil and some rosemary, and throw it in the oven at 375 until golden brown. Done! Baked sweet potato "fries." What's in that? Three ingredients, all of which came out of the ground. If you find yourself saying, "But wait, olive oil doesn't just come out of the ground," good for you! You're thinking critically about your food choices. Let's look at that a little closer. What's "in" extra-virgin olive oil? It's nothing more than the oil that's extracted from pressing olives. That certainly is as close to its natural state as possible.

Now, grab that bag of frozen sweet potato fries and look at the ingredients label. I'm willing to bet there's a ton of random ingredients in there that came out of a lab. Another good rule of thumb is if you can't pronounce it, put it back.

Of course, even in their natural state, some foods carry chemicals, hormones, and pesticides that would rival the nastiest processed food. Yes, I'm talking about the junk that nonorganic foods can bring to the party. These wreak havoc on your body and can lead to an unwanted spare tire.

For food to be certified organic it must meet strict criteria, a set of rules that govern how it's grown, stored, packaged, and shipped. While they vary somewhat in different countries, the standards generally forbid the use of synthetic chemicals, mandate that the grower use land that hasn't been touched by synthetic chemicals for at least three years, require separation from other nonorganic products, and require ongoing inspections to ensure all standards are being met.

These rules are in place to protect your health, but you're probably wondering how eating nonorganic food can make you fat. Let's quickly talk about your liver. It has two important jobs when it comes to weight loss: burning fat and filtering out harmful toxins. Nonorganic food is sprayed with chemicals or, in the case of meats and poultry, fed growth hormones. When you eat it, you're eating those chemicals and some of those hormones. If your liver is over-burdened trying to filter out all those harmful toxins, it can't focus on burning fat. Best solution? Give it a vacation. Take away the duty of filtering those poisons and it can become a fat-torching furnace.

Yes, I know it's more expensive to eat organic and if you have a large family it may seem unrealistic. But here's some good news: Not everything you eat has to be organic, and there are some easy rules to make it count when you do.

Meat, seafood, dairy, and fruits and veggies with edible or thin skins should all be organic. The thinner the skin (think strawberry), the more it will soak up chemicals. Ever taken a bite of celery and felt your lips and inside of your mouth tingling like someone just hosed you with bleach? It wasn't organic. Celery is 95 percent water and can transport a world of nasty chemicals into your body very quickly. The thicker the skin on your fruits and veggies (think avocado), the harder it is for pesticides to penetrate and the less important it is for it to be organic. That comes with an exception: If you're going to eat or use the peel or rind, like the zest of a lemon, for example, go organic.

Here's a fun cheat sheet that you can take with you to the grocery store. (This is also available for free at www.the30secondbody.com. Go print it out!)

The DIRTY Dozen Fruits and Veggies

(purchase only organic)

Apples	Lettuce
Bell peppers	Nectarines
Berries	Peaches
Celery	Pears
Cherries	Potatoes
Grapes	Spinach

The CLEAN Fifteen

(not *so* important to get organic)

Asparagus	Mango
Avocado	Mushrooms
Cabbage	Onions
Cantaloupe	Pineapple
Corn	Sweet peas
Eggplant	Sweet potatoes/ Yams
Grapefruit	Watermelon
Kiwi	

Remember, organic food may be more expensive than its non-organic counterpart, but it's a heck of a lot cheaper than a lifetime of medical bills. When it comes to your health, think about the big picture and commit to being healthy *for life*. Remember, you can pay at the grocery store or you can pay at the doctor's office. Eating healthfully may cost a few bucks more up front, but I promise it'll cost you a lot less in the long run!

#2 *Eat a Little Less*

"Duh!" you say? I know, it sounds simple. And it is. But it's still possible to get it wrong. Regardless of the latest diet craze, if you want to lose weight, you have to burn more calories in a day than you consume. I say that with a major caveat, which is that not all calories are created equal. For example, 1,600 calories of pizza and Cinnabons are not the same as 1,600 calories of vegetables. Good food makes you feel great. Bad food makes you feel terrible. Again, see #1 above.

In any event, I think you'll be relieved to know that you don't need to starve yourself (you don't get a prize for not eating; you just get hungry) or count calories to practice this principle. You can lose weight and still be an awesomely normal person who isn't waking up hungry in the middle of the night or measuring out protein grams on a scale. Who has time for that?!

Here's the first step: If your goal is to lose weight, stop eating when you feel about 80 percent full. What, you don't have a gauge on your belly? It's okay, just slow down and listen to your body. When you're about 80 percent full, you should feel well satiated, but not stuffed. Never eat to the point of being stuffed. You know that feeling after a meal where you take a big breath and exhale with slight audible exasperation? Yeah, you want to avoid that. Here are some easy tricks that will help. Again, you may think that this is *too* obvious, but if you're looking to lose some inches I'd be willing to bet that you're not practicing this with regularity. Just give it a shot and watch what happens.

- Take smaller portions.
- Drink a full glass of water before your meal.
- Drink a full glass of water after your meal.
- Use a smaller plate.
- Don't help yourself to seconds.
    - Wait 15 minutes before considering another helping. That urge to eat is most likely mental.
- Don't finish your entire meal.

That last one can be a doozy. I know a lot of us have issues with throwing out food. Some of it has to do with feeling like we have to get our money's worth, particularly at a restaurant that's served us the equivalent of two meals. To that I say, let it go. Do you really want to pay to make yourself fat?

And of course, a lot of it goes back to childhood. "Karen! Finish your plate or you're not getting up from the table," Mom would yell. "There are starving children all around the world!"

I get it. But it's time to come to terms with something. Eating every last bite on your plate isn't going to do a single thing to help people who are deprived of food. There are much better ways to address that issue. If it's something that's important to you, I recommend spending an hour researching how you can use your time and/or money to help and then take action. An hour should be all you need to get the ball rolling. Any more than that and you're likely slipping into a research black hole. Just take action in a meaningful way and stop guilting yourself into gaining weight. Deal?

And if you absolutely just cannot bring yourself to throw out what's left on your plate, package it up and make it into a different meal for tomorrow.

Another incredibly effective strategy is to slow down and fully enjoy your meals. When you're eating, eat. No distractions. Leave the TV off, put the computer to sleep, put down your phone, and actually be present during mealtimes. If you're fortunate enough to be dining with someone, enjoy their company.

I'm Italian. My extended family is very Italian. And though they're all wonderfully unique in their own ways (yes, even a little crazy . . . the best ones always are!), they have one thing in common: a zest for life. Regardless of what they have in the bank, they live life fully, taking their time to luxuriate in and be grateful for all things big and small. It's very inspiring and something you can model when it comes to eating. Take pleasure in your food, whether it's a meal that's been prepared for hours or a quick lunch on the go. Research has shown that people who practice periods of mindfulness tend to be happier overall. So you'll eat less *and* feel better, all without depriving yourself. Happy and lean? Not a bad combo.

But how can you be sure that there's a proper portion on your plate? I'm going to show you how to use a simple tool to control your calories and "measure" your food. You may be surprised to find that you already have it with you at all times and it won't cost you a dime!

#3 *Eat 5 Times Per Day*

Think breakfast, snack, lunch, snack, and dinner. Funny how that just so happens to fit in with most modern lives. If you work in an office or from home, are in school or on the road, you should be able to follow this five-times rule without it majorly disrupting your normal patterns of living. Breakfast, lunch, and dinner will be your biggest meals of the day, with your two snacks being a bit smaller.

So why eat five times per day? Simple: Food is what powers your metabolism ➔ Your metabolism is what provides energy to your body ➔ The faster your metabolism, the more calories you burn.

By eating clean, unprocessed foods throughout the day, you can rev up your metabolism and ignite your body's natural fat-burning process. Want:

- More energy?
- More strength?
- Hot body?
- Awesome sleep?

Think of your metabolism like a gas-powered engine that fuels your car in the dead of winter. Without fresh gas, the engine is going to putter out and the car will eventually stall. And when it does, your walk home is going to be very cold.

Just to be clear, when I say "eat five times a day" I am also saying "skipping meals is a fast track to fat!"

Say it with me: *"Skipping meals is a fast track to fat."*

Now keep repeating it like a mantra while I explain why.

My friend Deb and I met for lunch recently. It was around one in the afternoon and as we sat down, she started telling me how she'd been trying to lose weight for the last couple of months, but wasn't making any progress. She explained that her "weight loss plan" was more or less to work out occasionally, doing some long, slow (read: boring) cardio, and eat as little as possible. In fact, her turkey sandwich on a white roll with mayo, Sun Chips, and a Snapple were the first things she had eaten all day (quick quiz: What on that lunch tray is food as close to its natural state as possible? Answer: very little). "Dude," I said, "there's a reason you're not losing any weight. Look at how you're eating. Or more to the point, *not* eating."

Starve yourself and you'll lose weight, right? Au contraire!

When your body is deprived of food, it goes into a self-preservation mode where it begins to hold on to your current fat stores. Scientifically speaking, not eating triggers a stress response in your body, which releases cortisol, a hormone that stimulates hunger and cues the body to store fat. The next time you eat, it will store that food as fat, too. Why? Because your DNA is hardwired back to the days of our cave brothers and sisters and it remembers the dangers of going for days on end without food during times of scarcity.

Simply put: Your body is protecting itself.

It's one of the most amazingly resourceful things on the planet and it will go to war to ensure its survival. Ironically, the only loser in this war is, in fact, your body. So lay down your weapons and wave the white flag. It's time to surrender. Or, if you'd like to keep fighting, pick up a new weapon (a fork) and charge the battlefield (your kitchen)! If you feed your body a steady stream of smart, healthy foods in moderate portions, you'll ignite its natural fat-burning process and stay lean for life.

And finally, here's a no-brainer: When you eat five times per day, there's a far better chance that you're going to make better choices with each meal. Think about it. If you started your day with a bowl of oatmeal with fresh berries and walnuts or an egg omelet with veggies or a 30-Second Power Smoothie (the blueprint for which is at the end of this chapter), it's less likely that you're going to grab a chocolate chip muffin off that leftover breakfast tray in your office in midmorning. Depriving yourself because you think that's the key to weight loss is going to lead to what I call "holy hell I'm hungry" eating.

Come on. You know exactly what I'm talking about. At this point you're a little tired, a lot cranky, and just need to eat something, anything. You're not driven by smart eating principles, but autopiloted by hunger. Portion control? Whatever! Clean whole foods? Child, please! Bring on the drive-thru window at Taco Bell!

Listen, I've been there. Everything I've learned is from personal experience, both through the work I've done with myself and with people of all different backgrounds and body types. So let's climb aboard the Eat-Five-Times-Per-Day train and ride it all the way to Sexy Abs Town.

Eating five times a day isn't hard. You're going to start with breakfast and then eat just about every two and a half hours. I'd like you to eat breakfast before you leave the house in the morning, but if you work in an office and love eating at your desk, fine.

The day might look something like this:

Breakfast 7–8 A.M.
Egg omelet with sautéed veggies and avocado slices

Snack 10–10:30 A.M.
1 whole apple with a small handful raw, unsalted nuts

Lunch 12:30–1:30 P.M.

Kale salad with grilled salmon, unlimited green veggies, and quinoa

Snack 3:30–4:30 P.M.

Clean Power Smoothie

Dinner 6–7:30 P.M.

Broiled rosemary chicken with mashed sweet potatoes and oven-roasted broccoli

If you're a cop who works nights, like my brother-in-law Danny, this timetable probably isn't going to work for you. So use the example above as a suggested framework and adjust those hours according to your schedule. Your life. Your design. Just try to eat your first meal within an hour of waking and let that every-2½-hours principle guide the rest of your meals. You should be having your last meal of the day a minimum of 2½ hours before you go to bed. That will let your sleeping body focus its energy on recovery and restoration rather than digestion, allowing you to wake up fresh and energized. If you find yourself super-hungry in the time between dinner and bed, try sipping a cup of herbal tea before going back to the fridge. If your belly is still yelling at you, enjoy a half cup of plain Greek yogurt.

Whatever your schedule, eating this way will keep your metabolism burning like the calorie-torching furnace it was born to be.

#4 Pile On the Protein

Want to lose fat? How about building long, lean muscle? Any interest in improving your metabolism, powering your toughest workouts, and feeling fuller longer? You get the point. If you want all this and more, you need to make sure you're getting enough protein throughout the day. But here's an important fact: Your body can't store protein for later use. Once you've eaten it, it's either used to repair muscle tissue or passed out of the body. It's simply not possible to "load up" on protein in one shot. So inhaling a twenty-four-ounce rib-eye for breakfast and calling it a day isn't going to cut it. You need to replenish your protein stores consistently.

Whether the source is vegetarian or animal based, it should be on your plate at every meal. But not just any protein will do. You want to make sure it's lean, clean, and of the highest quality. So while a packaged deli meat slice may have a lot of protein, it doesn't fit the bill here as it's usually highly processed, filled with more than just the cut of meat (hello, nitrates and artificial flavorings!), and loaded with saturated fat (not *quite* as evil as was once believed to be, but still to be eaten in real moderation), which is something we'll get to shortly. The key to great health and lasting weight loss is to go for the highest-quality versions of everything you put in your body (see #1). The guide below, which appears in the upcoming keys as well, will help you decipher your best options.

Green Light—These are your best choices, so eat these the most.

- Eggs (whole or whites)
- Fish (wild, not farmed)
- Lean poultry (baked, grilled, roasted, steamed)
- High-protein grains (amaranth, bulgur, quinoa, etc.)
- Legumes (peas, beans, lentils)
- Nut butters (Read the label and find an option that has one ingredient: nuts. Crazy, but a lot of nut butters add sugar and salt. Totally unnecessary.)
- Raw nuts
- Pea, hemp, or whey protein (find one that's free of any artifi-

cial flavors or sweeteners, preservatives, or sugars. Go organic if possible, but if it's whey, make sure it's coming from cows not treated with rBGH, a nasty growth hormone)

Yellow Light—enjoy occasionally. Once a day is okay, but not with every meal.

- Cheese
- Fatty meats (Beef, pork, lamb. Go for lean cuts of grass-fed organic. Find a good butcher and get to know him or her really well. The guy at your local grocery store should be able to help point you in the direction of quality meats. Just tell him or her you want lean, grass-fed, organic.)
- Poultry skin

Red Light—avoid entirely, or at least eat as little as possible.

- Fast food (drive-thru burgers, Philly cheesesteaks, etc.)
- Fried fish and/or meats (Fish and chips, chicken-fried steak, any fried fish or fried meat options at a restaurant. Most chain restaurants use oils that are filled with trans fats [really bad, as they may not only raise your bad cholesterol, but can lower your good cholesterol as well]. They also tend to reuse their oil over and over again, which makes it more saturated [also, not the best thing] and honestly is just plain gross.)
- Processed meats (packaged bacon, deli meats, hot dogs, mass-produced sausage)

Now you know the good protein from the bad. But just how much is enough? This is really easy to calculate.

Hold up your hands and take a good look. These are the only

measuring tools you'll need to control your calories and gauge proper portion sizes for your body.

Men: Eat 2 palm-sized portions of lean protein with breakfast, lunch, and dinner

Women: Eat 1 palm-sized portion of lean protein with breakfast, lunch, and dinner

In case there's any confusion, for both men and women, a palm-sized portion is the thickness of your hand with the diameter measured from the base of your fingers to the bottom of your palm. And yes, some folks have particularly large or small hands when compared to their bodies, but on the whole our hands are proportionate to our overall body sizes. This method is simple and it works. Just give it a shot.

As for your two snacks per day, you're not going to be eating large meals for them (just look at the examples above in #3 for the rough size of the snacks you should eat) so you can ignore the palm principle. Just make sure that your snacks include some protein, whether in the form of nuts, protein powder in a shake, or a bit of lean chicken. You get the idea. And if you're freaking out right now because you want exact measurements and precise recipes, please relax. Listen to your body and proceed accordingly with total self-sufficiency. If after three weeks, you feel like you're not getting the results you want, maybe slim down the size of your snacks. Starving and feeling like you don't have enough energy? Dial them up a touch. Every *body* is different. Remember, this is all about *you* and should be fun!

Use the guide above as just that, a guide, and let that Refrigerator Phrase be a filter for your every bite: *good foods go bad* or *food as close to its natural state as possible.*

#5 Eat Carbs with Confidence

You've probably heard that you need carbohydrates in your diet. It's true. Carbs are one of three essential macro nutrients that your body needs to function properly (the other two are protein and fat—see above and below). But trying to decipher good carbs from bad can make your head spin faster than a Tilt-A-Whirl. And the more you google, the more confusing it gets. That, my friend, is not what this book is all about. This book is about clarity, simplicity, and results.

So, here's what you need to know: Eat carbs from unrefined, unprocessed food sources. Limit the others.

The former will break down and absorb slowly upon digestion, allowing you to maintain stable energy and blood sugar levels. They'll also keep you feeling fuller longer and help you stay lean. The latter break down and absorb quickly, which leads to more fat storage, energy crashes, and quicker bouts of hunger.

If you have a decent amount of weight to lose, limit your carb consumption to vegetables and fruits. Once you get lean and mean, you can start to incorporate nonveggie carbs back into your diet in moderate portions. Sounds severe, but if you want faster results, you've got to be willing to make a few minor sacrifices. Ask yourself whether the instant gratification you get from slamming down that slice of cake or plate of pasta or hunk of white bread is worth the regret and results that follow.

Ready to rock? Let's use the green, yellow, red light metaphor again:

Green Light (go ahead and eat):

- Fruits
- Legumes
- Vegetables
- Whole grains (amaranth, barley, buckwheat, bulgur, faro, quinoa, oatmeal, whole grain wheat flour, sprouted whole wheat)

Yellow Light (eat in limited amounts):

- Refined grains (processed cereals, white flour, white rice, pastas, any bread whose first ingredient is anything other than "whole grain wheat flour" or "sprouted whole wheat")

* Be careful of food packaging! Brands are very clever with their artwork and use phrases like "All Natural" or "Whole Wheat" or "Multigrain." Regardless of what the front-of-package design tries to tell you, the first ingredient on the label needs to be either *whole grain wheat flour* or *sprouted whole wheat.* If it's anything else, put it back and try again. Be sure to watch breads for added sugars. It'll be lurking back there on the ingredients label. Solid brands like Ezekiel and Food for Life are available nowadays in most grocery stores. Give them a try!

Red Light (seriously limit or, ideally, cut out altogether):

- Commercially mass-prepared baked goods (cakes, chips, cookies, crackers, doughnuts—these are almost always filled with really bad fats)

- Fried fast foods (french fries, onion rings, fried doughnuts, etc., from quick-service restaurants)
- Soda
- Processed sugar products (more on this later)

Fruit: Friend or Foe?

Some fruits are simple carbohydrates. Because of that, you may come across some "diet tip" that recommends avoiding fruit consumption to lose weight. This should set off alarm bells in your head. Yes, some fruits are simple carbohydrates that will break down and absorb quickly in the body. But regardless of its ranking on the glycemic index, whole fruit is packed with essential vitamins, minerals, and fiber that do a world of good for your body. In general, a principle that tells you not to eat fruit will likely lead to confusion and bad choices. "Expert Eddie told me not to eat fruit so, uh, I'm just gonna grab one of those diet bars from the vending machine." That's just crazy town! Overall, remember #3 (Eat 5 Times Per Day), and when it comes to fruit, eat up and ignore the fads!

It's pretty hard to get fat eating a ton of asparagus. When it comes to green vegetables, eat as much as you want! But if you're eating any other carb source, here's how much to portion with every meal.

Men: 1 fist-sized portion, max, with breakfast, lunch, and dinner

Women: Half of a fist-sized portion, max, with breakfast, lunch, and dinner

#6 *Eat More Vegetables*

When it comes to vegetables, forget the green, yellow, and red traffic lights. Go for greens, yellows, reds, oranges, purples, and every other conceivable color. Taste the rainbow, man! Most of us don't get enough vegetables, and that's a crying shame, as their value can't be overstated. Veggies are packed with nutrients that can set the stage for a fat-burning, fist-pumping party in your body. And guess what? There's nothing wrong with frozen vegetables. Yes, it would be great for you to eat fresh broccoli from your local farmer's market, but if that's too much of a logistical nightmare and it means you're instead going to go for a box of Rice-A-Roni, cut open a bag of frozen organic broccoli florets and go to town! It's easy to keep a few bags in your freezer for last-minute snack options.

You really can't eat too many veggies, but so you have a frame of reference of how much you should be eating at a minimum, roll up your sleeves and prepare your handy-dandy measuring tools.

Men: 2 fist-sized portions with breakfast, lunch, and dinner

Women: 1 fist-sized portion with breakfast, lunch, and dinner

While it's better to eat whole vegetables, some folks find it hard to eat enough veggies every day. If you're one of them, it's better to get the nutrients from a supplement than not at all. Always remember, supplements are meant to do just that: supplement your daily diet. Strive to get your nutrients from whole foods first. Then, and only then, supplement with products that are derived from whole, organic foods.

By Any Means Necessary

My favorite green supplement is called *Amazing Grass Green Superfood*. It's a powder made from organic green foods and can be mixed into any beverage. I just mix it with water. Again, it shouldn't replace your efforts to eat the real thing. But I promise not to judge if you need a little help in the form of powdered organic greens from time to time!

#7 Feast on Fats

Like proteins and carbs, your body needs fat. No, fat won't make you fat. And no, cutting fat out of your diet completely will not help you lose fat. In fact, it can sabotage your weight loss goals. The thing to understand is that not all fats are created equal. There are three types: unsaturated fats (good guys), saturated fats (kind of bad, mostly misunderstood guys), and trans fats (evil villains).

The kinda, sorta bad guys and really bad guys can clog your arteries, increase your risk of heart disease, raise your bad cholesterol levels (LDL), and wreak havoc on your metabolism, causing you to gain weight. What makes trans fats particularly bad is that not only can they do all of the above, but they can actually lower your good cholesterol levels as well. Saturated fat is found in animal products such as meat and high-fat dairy, so you want to limit your intake of those. For a long time, we've been told that saturated fats should be avoided. As it turns out, that is too simplistic—they should not, in fact, be avoided entirely.

It can get a little complicated. So let's keep this simple: Remember rule #1 *above all* and be mindful with your saturated fat intake, even when it's coming from a source that's unprocessed and as close to its natural state as possible, like organic grass-fed beef. Now, saturated fats are *also* found in hydrogenated products like margarine, certain crackers, cookies, and chips. Skip those. Read labels and be on the lookout for the word *hydrogenated*. If you see that, just put it back on the shelf and keep on truckin'.

The good guys, on the other hand, can actually help reduce your risk of heart disease and lower cholesterol levels. How much is enough? Here's the thing: If you're filling your plate with the suggested portion sizes of clean, lean proteins I'm talking about at breakfast, lunch, and dinner, you're likely already getting enough fats. But let's say you're adding *additional* good fats like, say, avocado, olive oil, nut butters, etc., to a meal or having them with a snack. Here's how much to portion:

Men: 2 thumb-sized portions with any given meal
Women: 1 thumb-sized portion with any given meal

#8 Drink More Water. Drink Fewer Calories

This is a biggie. Most people go about their day in a state of mild dehydration. That's a bad thing if you want to avoid muscle weakness, brain fatigue, and organ failure. And I think we'd all like to avoid organ failure. But your interest here is in losing weight. And for that reason alone, you should start drinking more water. Half your body weight in ounces to be precise. So, if you weigh 160 pounds, you should be drinking 80 ounces of water each day.

Why? Well, in addition to helping to transport and absorb nutrients, digest food, prevent constipation, and regulate body temperature, water can also help with portion control. Downing a glass of water before a meal helps you feel fuller, which in turn will curb the likelihood that you'll overeat.

Super-complicated, right?

Making sure you drink enough water is one of the easiest and single best things you can do for your body. I want you to look at a glass of clear, pure water and imagine your body, inside and out, just as clear and pure. The visualization alone is enough to give you a little rush of happy vibes. Now drink up!

How to Drink Enough Water

- Buy a nice-looking bottle and carry it around with you. Pick something that's BPA-free. I reuse a glass water bottle. Easy peasy!
- Set a glass of water on your nightstand or next to your bed and drink it when you first wake up.
- Drink a glass before every meal.
- Drink a glass after every meal.
- Add fresh fruit. Lemons, limes, kiwis, cherries, etc. Slice up whatever fruit you like and toss it in. It'll flavor your water without weighing you down.

How can you tell if you're drinking enough when you don't have a measuring cup at the office? Simple! At home, measure out how many ounces it takes to fill your water bottle (if it doesn't already tell you on the side). Let's say it takes 20 ounces to fill your bottle and you need to drink 80 ounces per day. You now know that you should drink about four of those bottles before you hit the sack.

Another quick tip if you forget your bottle. At home, measure out 10 ounces of water and count how many normal swallows it takes you to finish. Jot that number down so you'll remember it. Measure at home; drink anywhere!

Drinking more water is half the battle. Cutting out the calorie-bomb beverages is the other. Say it with me: Soda is evil. Pure evil. A Big Gulp has about 500 calories in one cup—500! And I'm sorry, but I've got some bad news for you zero-calorie, no-sugar diet soda sippers. It's no better. You've just swapped the sugar for artificial sweeteners, which are chemical catastrophes just waiting to destroy your waistline and overall health.

And what about sports drinks? Are you training for a triathlon? If yes, go for it after you work out. No? Then skip the sports drink and toss some lemon slices in water to rehydrate after a workout! Most sports drinks have far too many calories for the recreational athlete. And the "next-gen" zero-calorie versions? Just like with diet soda, they're packed with unnecessary additives. Remember, keep the stuff you put in your body unprocessed and as close to its natural state as possible.

Commercial orange juice, apple juice, other fruit juice, and those fake fruit drinks all have the same thing in common: an abundance of gut-busting sugar. Drinking juice is not the same thing as eating whole fruit. Don't be fooled by the cute marketing campaign on the front of that carton of OJ telling you that one glass gives you a full day's serving of fruit. Whole fruits have vitamins and minerals and heart-healthy fiber. When you eat fruit, you're getting all of that goodness. Most packaged fruit juices, meanwhile, are stripped of all the good stuff, leaving nothing more than a glass of liquid sugar. If you're craving fruit juice, eat the real thing.

#9 *Pump the Brakes on Sugar*

A lot of experts will tell you unequivocally that sugar is the devil and that you should avoid it at all costs. And there's no getting around it: It's bad for your health and waistline. But saying to avoid it entirely is probably a recipe for failure. Denying ourselves something that we love usually leads to a binge or at least a sense of deprivation. And you don't want either of those. You want a hot body and healthy, happy life. So here's the rule of thumb: Go easy on unnatural sugar. That is, don't worry about the sugars in fruits and vegetables (natural sugars) but pump the brakes as often as you can when it comes to candy, soda, cakes, table sugar, and the like. Less than you're eating now is a great start.

If you have a significant amount of weight to lose, I would recommend cutting refined, processed sugars from your diet entirely for twenty-one days and then revisiting your relationship with them a little at a time. This cold turkey approach won't be easy, but by the end of the twenty-first day, your cravings and taste for sugar will be significantly lower, if not entirely gone. Make it a challenge and take it head-on!

The Sugar Trap

Everyone knows that sugar tastes good. But the more of it we eat, the more our palate becomes accustomed to that sweet taste and the more we begin to crave it in all the foods we eat. Food manufacturers know that making their products sweeter will keep us coming back for more. That's what the evaporated cane juice and high-fructose corn syrup are doing in your processed foods (all the more reason to avoid processed foods—see Key #1!). We can't really blame the food marketers though—they're just giving us what we've come to want. So let's vote with our dollars. Cut down on your addiction to sugar and hypersweetened foods and we just might encourage a change in the way mass-prepared food is made. Hey, a guy can dream, right?

#10 *Treat. Don't Cheat.*

I'm going to say this straight out of the gate. I don't believe in cheat days. Some people swear by them. Me? Not so much. In the big picture and not some crash-diet mentality, I think they are a recipe for failure. First of all, whom exactly are you cheating? This is your life. You're in charge. I want you to feel empowered, not like you're hiding some shady behavior.

When you think about enjoying the things you love as cheating, you create a mindset that you're doing something wrong. You're not doing *anything* wrong. You're making choices. What you have to decide is whether the choices you're making are in line with your overall goals. Allowing "cheat days" into your vocabulary and life also sets up a binge mentality, which goes against the idea of moderation, which is one of the keys to success here. Deny yourself all week long and then go hog wild on Thursdays? That could lead to overindulging in calorie bombs that destroy all your hard work. And can you honestly tell me that even with a cheat day, you're not going to have a little somethin' somethin' at that spur-of-the-moment happy hour?

So then what's the solution? The 80/20 Rule.

It's a simple philosophy: 80 percent of your food choices are healthy and 20 percent are indulgences. You may have heard of this since it's a pretty common piece of advice, but I want you to think about it in the context of Key #3 (Eat 5 Times Per Day).

As you know, you're now going to eat five times each day (breakfast, snack, lunch, snack, dinner). The 80/20 rule allows you to treat yourself to the things you love every day, be it chocolate, ice cream, wine, beer, booze, or whatever else you fancy. That's right. Every. Day.

Here's your move: If you want to treat (not cheat) yourself, then you're going to simply replace one of your snacks for a treat. Ooey gooey cookie? Fresh baked doughnut? Neapolitan pizza? You can have it. You're simply going to take one snack out of rotation that day in exchange for a treat. Makes sense, right? It's super-easy and prevents you from feeling like you're denying yourself things you love. *That* sounds like a diet. *This* sounds like a life.

Here's what it might look like:

Breakfast **7–8 A.M.**
Snack **10–10:30 A.M.**
Lunch **12:30–1:30 P.M.**
~~Snack **3:30-4:30 P.M.**~~
Dinner **6–7:30 P.M.**
Treat **Ice Cream**

The key with this is to exercise moderation with your indulgences. This is the only time I'm going to ever ask you to examine calories. Don't obsess but be aware of what you're eating by checking out the calories per serving *and* the number of servings per package. A package of cookies may tell you it's only 200 calories, but after further examination you see that's per serving. And a suggested serving is two cookies, but there are four in the pack. Keep your eyes open, you little detective, you, and you won't be fooled.

Some mistake the notion of the 80/20 rule to mean that as long as they're eating healthfully throughout the day, they can pound a beast of a dessert with no consequences. I'm not here to judge. I'm here to educate, and if you really want to lose weight and get lean for life, you need to get a handle on this. Ideally, you want to keep your daily treat to around 200 calories. To give you an idea, a standard pack of Reese's Peanut Butter Cups is 210 calories and a glass of wine is around 125. Is it going to kill you to go over your 200 allotment by a few points? Of course not. Just be mindful and keep it in check.

For you salty-tooth folks, the same principle applies. Want that bag of chips? Keep your portion to around 200 calories and cut out one of your snacks that day.

But let's say you want to indulge a little bigger. You've got a birthday party coming up and you know there's going to be amazing drinks and cake. You can save up your treats for a few days and go all out on, say, an 800-calorie lovefest. I wouldn't really go more than three or four days max on this, though, because then it starts to morph into that "cheat day" mentality. Just remember on the weeks you do this, that it's an extra-special indulgence!

The Three-Bite Rule

Don't know the full calorie count or serving size of what's calling to you from the dessert buffet? Here's a little trick I use when I really want to indulge, but don't want to blow all the hard work I've put in on my body. I use it mostly for desserts, but it can really be used for any food.

It's simple: Limit yourself to three bites.

The first bite satisfies your psychological desire and is usually just as satisfying as you'd hoped it would be. Take your time chewing it. Really enjoy this bite.

The second bite is still pretty darn good, but if you really pay attention, it's not quite as good as the first, right? But chew and swallow—this bite will help satisfy your appetite.

The third bite is the capper. It's not going to taste any better after that second bite, so choose to end the experience here. It's like leaving a really fun party before things get sloppy.

Here's the thing: The Three-Bite Rule ain't gonna work if you just mindlessly inhale whatever's sitting in front of you or take three enormously large bites. The key is to stay mindful. No need to get weird. Just be present while you're eating and really enjoy the treat. You may not even want the third bite.

Whatever's left over, trash it. And don't feel bad. We already reviewed this. You're not going to guilt yourself into weight gain anymore.

#11 Raise a Glass?

Oh the dreaded A-word. You want to know if you can still indulge in alcohol, right? Here's the potentially painful answer: yes, but only so much as your 80/20 (treat don't cheat) rule allows.

Sorry, but that's the long and the short of it. Alcohol has a ton of empty calories, not to mention all the sugar and preservatives in any mixers you might be adding. And in all fairness, liquor whittles away at our better judgment, which often leads to really poor food choices. When are you usually getting tipsy? At night. Where? At a bar or restaurant or dinner party (or in your own kitchen) where you also have access to food. What happens when you're totally plastered?

Your principles and goals are far more likely to get flung out the window in favor of a bar pizza or another bottle of wine.

If you know you have a drinks meeting or party or something that will involve cocktails, plan strategically and save up a few of your treats by cutting down on daily snacks. I wish there were a magic answer for this topic. Trust me. I love a good adult beverage as much as the next guy. But if your goal is to cut your belly fat, then you need to curb the drinking. In the long run, your mind, body, and business will be better for it.

Tips for staying in control around alcohol:

- Order water or seltzer in a rocks glass with a twist of lime and toss in a red straw. It looks enough like a cocktail for you not to seem like a buzzkill.
- Drink sllllowwwly.
- Have a glass of water after every drink. And drink that glass of water sllllowwwly.
- Order clear spirits with no mixers. Tequila neat or on the rocks with a twist of lime is seriously low-cal and packs a powerful punch.

#12 *Cleanses and Juices and Fasts. Oh My!*

I've done just about every cleanse out there. I've juiced and fasted, and I can tell you that there is *some* merit to *some* of it. But not as a replacement to a healthy whole-foods-based eating lifestyle. Remember, fads are, by definition, unsustainable. Yes, you will lose weight on a "cleanse" where you're only taking in liquids for any number of days. And yes, you may "reset" your palate if you've been going hog wild lately. But the minute you start eating food again, your weight will swing back up to where you started, and possibly higher.

So don't let some celebrity who "has that glow" convince you that you need to try Dr. So-and-So's new cleansing revolution. For one thing, Ms. Deweyface was likely just done up by a $300 per hour makeup artist who put the final moisturizing touches on her face mere seconds before she stepped in front of the camera on an expertly lit set. For another, she likely holds a financial interest in Dr. So-and-So's company. I encourage you to read between the lines.

All that said, don't confuse a commercial cleanse with throwing delicious whole foods in a blender and drinking them down before you leave the house—that is, a Clean Power Smoothie (see the end of this chapter). Blending and drinking good ingredients instead of chewing and swallowing isn't the same thing as subsisting on spicy lemonade for a week. When you blend, you're getting the whole food, fiber and all. The blender is just breaking the food down for easier digestion and absorption.

Are you going to individually eat a cup of berries, big handful of spinach, spoonful of almond butter, scoop of protein powder, and iced green tea for breakfast? Probably not. But throw it all into a blender and you have yourself an incredibly nutritious and surprisingly delicious meal that'll whittle your waistline and give you more nutrients in a glass than most people in your office probably get in a week. (And even if you're not a big fan of spinach, I would implore you to try it just once! I think you'll be pleasantly surprised.)

Let's Recap

Here's what should be on your plate at breakfast, lunch, and dinner:

- High-quality protein
  - Guys: 2 palms. Gals: 1 palm.
- Veggies
  - Guys: 2 fists. Gals: 1 fist.
  - Can't do it? If necessary, try a powdered supplement like the one mentioned in Key #6.
- If adding a carb beyond a veggie source (like grains)
  - Guys: 1 fist max. Gals: ½ fist max.
- Healthy fat
  - Guys: 2 thumbs. Gals: 1 thumb.
  - Remember, you likely already have enough fat on your plate by this point from your lean protein source, but if you'd like to add more or are including healthy fats in a snack, keep it to the serving size mentioned in Key #7.
- Zero-calorie, zero-processed-additives beverage
  - Preferably water.
- Snacks
  - These should be smaller than the other three meals and include some form of lean, clean protein and preferably a veggie or fruit.

Hungry yet? Awesome! I hope you now realize that nutrition tastes good and that "diets" no longer have a place in your life. Grab some grub (five times a day) and keep it clean.

As promised, here's the template for a Clean Power Smoothie. There are tons of potential combos that you can bring to life right in your own kitchen, so get creative!

6 STEPS TO BUiLD A BETTER SMOOTHiE

1. Start with a veggie. About 1–2 large handfuls.
   - Flower, fruit, or seed vegetable (artichoke, cucumber, peas, pumpkin, squash, tomato, etc.)
   - Stem or leaf vegetable (asparagus, broccoli, celery, chard, kale, rhubarb, spinach, etc.)
   - Root vegetable (beet, carrot, lotus root, radish, sweet potato, etc.)
2. Add fruit. About 1–2 small handfuls.
   - Citrus fruit (grapefruit, kumquat, lemon, lime, mandarin, orange, etc.)
   - Deciduous fruit (apple, apricot, cherry, figs, nectarine peach, pear, plum, quince, etc.)
   - Vine fruit (berries, grapes, kiwi, passion fruit, pitaya, etc.)
3. Toss in a protein powder. 1–2 scoops.
   - Whey (rBGH-free)
   - Hemp
   - Pea
   - Rice

4. Layer in a nut, nut butter, or seed. About 1–2 thumb-sized portions.
   - Raw almond, cashew, peanut, walnut, etc., or the butter version of these (just make sure the only ingredient on the jar is the nut, nothing more)
   - Chia seeds, flaxseeds, hemp seeds, etc.
5. Add a zero-calorie or very-low-calorie liquid.
   - Water
   - Iced black coffee
   - Iced green tea
   - Unsweetened almond milk
6. Blend and top it off.
   - If you'd like to give your smoothie a little visual flair after blending and make it feel like more of a meal, sprinkle any of these on top:
     - Crushed or slivered nuts
     - Cinnamon
     - Coconut
     - Fresh berries
     - Goji berries
     - Oats

Here's an example of one of my favorites.

Super Berry Detox

- Step 1: 1 large handful of spinach
- Step 2: 1 small handful of frozen mixed organic berries (straw-berries, blueberries, raspberries, and blackberries; usually what's in a single bag in the freezer at my health food store)
- Step 3: 1 scoop of vanilla whey protein powder

- Step 4: 1 large teaspoon raw peanut butter
- Step 5: Iced green tea
- Step 6: Blend and top with a small handful of fresh blue-berries
- Step 7: Enjoy

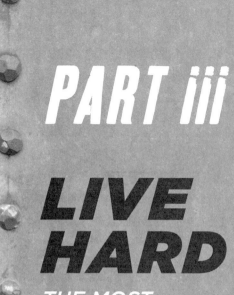

PART iii

LIVE HARD

THE MOST
IMPORTANT PART
OF THE BOOK

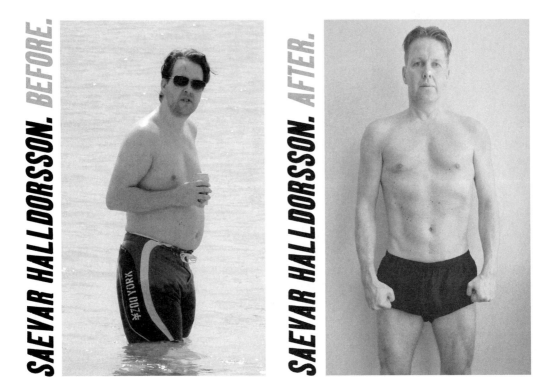

SAEVAR HALLDORSSON. BEFORE.

SAEVAR HALLDORSSON. AFTER.

"I was a part of the test group for *The 30-Second Body*. When I started it, I was overweight, unhappy, and depressed after a recent divorce. I had hit an emotional, mental, and physical wall and knew I had to change something in my life.

"I signed up as a desperate attempt to just do something. Honestly, I regretted it immediately and came up with hundreds of excuses for how to get out. I decided to show up for the first class, go through it, and then tell Adam that this was too tough for me and never come back. I hadn't even gone to the first class and this was already my mindset.

"First, he put us through a fitness test and had us write down all our reps for six exercises. It was the hardest thing I had ever done. I had to pause every five seconds to catch my breath, but Adam's positive encouragement pulled me through the exercises. After class he told me that I had done really well and that he looked forward seeing me the next day. My chance to bail out was gone and I forced myself to show up.

"In the second class I was still taking a break every five seconds, but sometimes I could go ten seconds straight. That may not seem like a lot, but to me that was 100 percent improvement and I could actually feel my stamina and energy getting better. I decided right then and there to commit 110 percent and fully adopt Adam's motto, 'Eat Clean. Train Dirty. Live Hard.' That night I did a Pantry Raid, getting rid of all the garbage in my fridge and cabinets and began eating only natural, unprocessed food.

"Getting off the sugar roller coaster and carb train was hard the first two weeks, but the workouts helped tremendously with the transition. Two weeks in, I was sleeping better, feeling better, and had a much more positive outlook on life than when I began.

"When we took our second fitness test, I looked at my numbers and saw that they had more than tripled on all six exercises. Something clicked in my head, and I was more determined than ever before.

"I saw it through to the very end, improving every single day, and stand here now a totally changed man. My stamina and energy are through the roof; I get compliments all the time; I'm no longer unhappy or depressed and, my God, just look at the photos. It's crazy to think that guy with the beer can was actually me. But I'm proud of where I came from. Without that journey, I wouldn't be the strong, confident man I am today. And as Adam always says, you're stronger than you think."

UNDERSTAND THE PROBLEM

WHAT'S BEEN STOPPING YOU FROM HAVING the body of your dreams? Was it the wrong plan? Maybe. A bad diet? Perhaps. But if you'd heard of clean eating before and were at some point following a decent exercise plan, what gives? There's something much bigger and more impactful holding you back and it's been growing inside you since you were a child.

It's your inability to take full responsibility and maintain consistency.

Yikes! Harsh, I know. But it's not entirely your fault. You've been conditioned to fail. I talked about this in the introduction, but it bears repeating. Since you were a child, companies with a lot of marketing dollars have told you that you can have anything you want with practically no effort at all. It's not a conspiracy. It's business. And the messaging is relentless.

Get washboard abs in five days!

Become a multimillionaire after one weekend seminar!

Achieve international stardom overnight!

Lose twenty pounds in one week with a new secret miracle pill!

There are endless variations, but they all have the same exact message: Get *ANYTHING* you want *IMMEDIATELY* with *ZERO* effort.

I call it Lottery Mindset Marketing. It plays to our "get-rich-quick" susceptibility. I've fallen prey to it more times than I care to admit. Who wouldn't? Can you honestly tell me that you would prefer to work your butt off for something if you could have it with no effort whatsoever? Companies know this and use it to sell you stuff. And if your mind is fed the same message over and over again, it's going to eventually accept it as truth and direct you to act accordingly, for better or worse.

Before we dive into fixing that little problem, there's something you should know about me. I'm nothing special. Yes, I do believe I'm great, but it's the same greatness that's inside *you*. At the end of the day there's nothing that makes me radically more exceptional than anyone else. I could easily be that friend you grew up with or your cousin that you see around the holidays. In fact, to a lot of people, that's *exactly* who I am. I'm just a guy. To this day, much to the chagrin of my team, I refuse to set up a Facebook fan page or make my profile private. People who want to connect send me a friend request just like they would for that guy they met at their friend's party the other weekend. You can click through my photos and see shots of me at my little cousin's birthday party or hanging out at the beach and doing other stuff that might qualify as "fancy." My aunt Cookie swears someone's going to show up at my house one day with a kooky grin and a few screws missing. It's cool. I'll invite them in for a barbecue.

The point is that I'm just like you in a great number of ways. But I have one driving mission: to *help* you live a healthy, happy, active life. Pretending to be some untouchable celebrity isn't going to help. It's actually one of my biggest pet peeves.

But there is something unique that people comment on time and time again that I can't ignore. It's my eternal optimism and knack for "just doing things" rather than endlessly talking about or overthinking them.

Over the years I've given this a lot of thought. Why do I believe that I can *just do things,* and what makes me stick to the things I set my mind to until I achieve them?

I blame my parents.

Seriously. Since I was little they never once made me believe that I was limited in any area of my life. To be clear, I'm not talking about being coddled or told I was a special snowflake. Far from it. I had my butt handed to me in that old-school take-no-crap kind of way more times than I care to remember. What my parents did was lead by example.

When I was little, I watched them buy a small family business, only to find out that it wasn't just seriously in debt, but bankrupt. To make a very long story short, after years of dedication and sacrifice, they turned it into a successful multimillion-dollar cornerstone of their community. It didn't happen overnight, and it sure didn't happen because they won the lottery. Their focus, hard work, and consistency delivered the results.

They showed me and told me that if there was anything I wanted to do, I could do it. And it never felt like a lesson in an after-school special because, honestly, it wasn't. They were incredibly young and just doing what they needed to do. But the message came across loud and clear in both word and action. They kind of Mr. Miyagi'd me, didn't they? Their daily teachings not only conditioned me with the best tools for success, but made me mostly impervious to that Lottery Mindset Marketing I was talking about. You may fool me once (hey, we're all susceptible!), but I can see through the BS. Try and tell me that miracles happen overnight—I've always known better. So, Mom and Dad, as I'm sure you're reading this for the seventeenth time, thank you, again.

So what about you? What if you didn't have Pete and Gail Rosante for parents? What if you got conditioned by that Lottery Mindset Marketing and/or worse, your family sometimes dropped fun statements like "You better marry rich," or "Oh no, you could never do that" or "You'll never be as thin as your sister"? If that's bringing up some hard personal stuff right now, I'm sorry. We all have our history. And while we can't change the past, we can sure as hell work in the present to make tomorrow un-freaking-real.

And guess what? You now have me as a friend. As long as you're willing to do your fair share of the work, I'm going to help you. You already have a clear plan to move and feed your body. Now I'm giving you a plan to train your mind so that not only will you stick to your six-week fitness program and clean eating lifestyle, but you will in fact take your entire life to the next level.

Let's get after it!

9 KEYS TO A LiMiTLESS LiFE

#1 *Quit the Blame Game*

Now that you know where your negative conditioning may come from, it's time to take full ownership of your life. I'm talking 100 percent responsibility. Nothing less will do. This may sound intimidating, but think about it for a second. If you take total responsibility for your life, you wield total power over it. Even those little (and sometimes major) things that happen throughout the day that seem to be out of your control are under your thumb when you decide how to respond to them. It's not complicated and doesn't have to cost you a dime. It's nothing more than a decision. And when you make that decision, you can truly live to the fullest. You can *live hard*.

It's not going to happen overnight. Again, this isn't a magic trick. It's also not an impossible or backbreaking task. It's just the power of consistency. Over time, many of us developed the habit of blaming others for the state of our lives. "Ugh! These soda sizes are just out of control! They're making me so fat." "I don't have the time to work out. I'm chained to a desk ten hours a day."

Dude. Stop.

That soda didn't climb into your hand and pour itself down your throat. Deciding to buy and drink it was your choice, as was the decision to go to bed late, snooze the alarm until you had to dash around your house like a crazy person, throw on some clothes, grab a bagel, and make it to the office just in time, instead of getting up an hour earlier to work out and eat a healthy breakfast. The first step toward positive change is accepting complete and total responsibility for our lives and the choices we make.

From this moment forward, every time you catch yourself shifting blame to someone or something else, you're going to stop and say to yourself, "I am in control of my life. My choices in this moment shape my realities in the next. I accept full responsibility."

This is going to take practice. And it may honestly feel a little corny at first. Be patient with yourself. If you play the blame game a lot, this may feel odd, physically uncomfortable even. But with enough practice it will become second nature and can take your body and your life to the next level.

Now, deep down we know that poor choices aren't going to help us get where we want to be. Then why do we make them and how do we go about making different ones? First, we need to wake up.

#2 Become a Track Star

At the end of the day, our lives are the net result of our habits. Habits are nothing more than behaviors that have become ingrained over time by the choices we make on a daily basis. The problem is that most of us aren't even aware of the choices we're making. It's like we're bumbling around on autopilot. How many times have you walked into your office's kitchen and grabbed a brownie off that leftover-snack tray? You gobbled it down only to regret it moments later (and I'm betting it wasn't even a very good brownie!). Why did you do it?

Sometimes you eat breakfast, healthy or not. Other times you don't. Lunch might be something from wherever the group is going or that you pulled out of your freezer that morning, all most likely options out of line with your desire to get in great shape. Why?

You're in a bit of credit card debt. Nothing major, but you'd like to clean it up and buy an apartment. Yet you spend money like it's going out of style. Again, why?

Because you're not thinking. You're just going about the day with a routine that's been populated with bad habits. Well, ignorance thrives in darkness, so the very first thing you're going to do is track your behavior and shine a bright light on all of your choices.

For one week, *starting right now,* you're going to write down every single thing you put into your body, liquid or solid. You can carry around a little pad and pen or just keep a note in your phone. When I say everything, I mean *everything*. We have a tendency to assume the little things don't count. From the oatmeal with berries and walnuts that you had for breakfast to the bite-size Kit Kat you grabbed off your coworker's desk to the Diet Coke you "snuck" in your lunch meeting and the bottle and a half of water you drank at your desk. No matter what it is, if you ingested it, write it down.

Exactly one week from now, review it. Tally up your wins (eating and drinking clean + doing your workouts each day) and losses (skipping meals and/or eating and drinking in a way that doesn't match up to my favorite phrases—*good foods go bad* and *food as close to its natural state as possible*—and skipping workouts). Take a good look and ask yourself, "How'd I do?"

Continue to track the same behaviors for another two weeks (three total), reviewing your performance at the end of each week. Breaking it down into one-week increments serves two purposes:

1) It allows your mind to settle into a totally doable framework (it's only a week!) and 2) it doesn't allow enough time to pass that this exercise gets away from you (again, it's only a week!).

Notice that I'm not asking you to do anything more than track your behavior. The brilliant thing about tracking is that you'll likely notice changes without having to do anything else just yet. It's almost too easy. The mere act of writing things down makes you stop and think about what you're doing, which in turn increases the likelihood that you'll make decisions in line with your goals of getting a lean, healthy body.

And why three weeks total? Some people say it takes twenty-one days to make or break a habit. I haven't found any hard science to back this up, but I have seen it work with myself and clients. So give it a shot!

Showing You the Money

I said this chapter could help you in every area of your life. We're obviously talking about losing weight and getting toned, but I want to prove to you the universal power of tracking with a story about my friend Kevin. Years ago, he was looking to pay off his student loans and get out from under what was for him a boatload of credit card debt. He had a pretty good job where he was making nice cash, but he always had a bit more month at the end of the money than money at the end of the month. So I had him track his expenses the exact same way I'm asking you to track your diet.

Yes, he was blowing money at bars and on a few bigger purchases, which he knew, but what he really exposed were the little things. The daily large iced coffee at Starbucks; a grab-and-go lunch with an approximate daily total of $16; and a bunch of other seemingly inconsequential expenses that he didn't "count." At the end of those three weeks, without doing anything other than tracking, he cut those expenses to less than a third by making coffee and lunch at home, cutting out a few other fairly small cash drains, scaling back on the trips to the bar, and stopping what he came to realize was his compulsive purchasing of songs on iTunes.

He then reallocated that money to savings and at the end of the month would dump it on one credit card with the highest interest rate, while paying the minimum on his other cards. Before long, he paid off that one card and set his sights on the next one, finding ways to continue saving a bit more here and there. Sure, he fell off on occasion, but for the most part he stayed the course, and when he reflexively went to open his wallet for something, he began to pause and give it more thought. And the small strides he made along the way encouraged him to stick with it. After a little over three years, my man was debt-free and turned all that money he had been paying toward debt into savings. Now, three years may seem like a really long time, but you have to realize he had been living with what he felt was an insurmountable pile of debt for almost ten years with no end in sight. If he can use tracking to turn around his finances in a relatively short amount of time, you can use it to turn around your body!

#3 Understand How and Why Goals Work

I've always liked new sneakers. I mean, *really* liked them. Since I was little, there were few things that would give me a bigger thrill than the smell of a brand-new pair of kicks. A funny thing would happen (and still does) when I'd set my sights on a specific pair of sneakers: I'd start to see that very pair *everywhere*. Of all the shoes that Reebok makes, I would see the same style and color nearly everywhere I looked. The first time I noticed this I swear I thought I was going crazy. It was like the universe was conspiring to give everyone a pair of Pumps but me.

Obviously that wasn't the case.

The sneakers were always there. I just wasn't paying attention.

Some people call it the Law of Attraction or the Secret. That's all just fancy talk for *focus*. When your mind focuses on something, it becomes highly attuned to that thing. Find yourself fiending for a trip to Mexico and you suddenly see ads for Mexico everywhere you look. Discover a hairstyle that you love and voilà, it seems like it's in all the magazines! Your mind focused on something specific and your eyes opened to it. *This is why goal-setting works*.

If you get crystal clear about what it is you want, your mind will focus on it and open your eyes to the possibility of making it a reality in your life. But just focusing on it won't make it happen. You're not going to sit in a room staring at a wall and will your way to a great body. You have to take action.

#4 Set Goals the Easy Way

People overcomplicate this. I swear there are more books, programs, and weekend seminars on goal-setting than there are people actually achieving their goals. There's no need for this to be difficult. My process is simple and it's been working for me since I was a teenager.

Grab a pen and some paper right now. I'm serious. I want you to do it right this second, not at the end of the chapter or later today. You start building the habit of taking immediate action *right now*.

Mark this page, set the book down, and get a pen and paper. I promise this won't take long.

1. **SIT:** Settle into a distraction-free zone with a pen and some paper. No phone, computer, people, etc. Put your phone in another room.

2. **PONDER:** Think about what you want from your entire life. Consider every area, not just fitness. Trust me; knowing what you want from your *entire* life will help you stick to your fitness goals. Plus, a sure road to unhappiness is focusing very heavily on just one single aspect of your life (for most people it's career) and letting the other stuff fall out of mind.

   The chart below is something I use to make sure I'm considering every area that I think is important and contributes to my total happiness. I call it *Life360*. Feel free to scratch out some of these categories and insert ones that make more sense for you. Or if this all resonates, use it as is. This is a highly personal exercise and should reflect *you*.

Life360

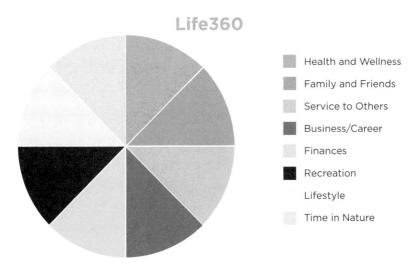

- Health and Wellness
- Family and Friends
- Service to Others
- Business/Career
- Finances
- Recreation
- Lifestyle
- Time in Nature

3. **BRAINSTORM:** Give these areas some thoughtful consideration. Do not get sidetracked. I repeat: It's important that you

put your phone in another room and be in a distraction-free zone so that if and when you hit a wall in your brainstorming, you don't default to fiddling on your phone or with something else in procrastination.

4. **WRITE:** At the top of a fresh sheet of paper, write down your categories. Under each category, start writing about *what* you want. Think about *why* you want it. Think about how you'll *feel* when you get there. This doesn't need to be a Pulitzer Prize–winning piece of literature and there are no wrong answers. Just let the thoughts from inside your head flow through the pen and onto the paper. Under Health and Wellness, do you want to lose weight? Do you want to handle stress better? Do you want more energy? Write it all down.

5. **BREAK:** When you're done, get up and grab a drink of water. Use the bathroom if you need to, but no other pit stops. Stay away from your phone.

6. **RESUME:** Come back to the paper and read what you've written for each category.

7. **EDIT:** There's probably some overlap in a few of your thoughts. Condense your desires for each category into more specific statements. It's okay if they're a bit broad at first, like "I want to be healthy."

8. **REFINE:** Further edit the results above into even more specific, actionable statements that begin with the powerful phrase "I am." So, "I want to be healthy" turns into "I am losing 20 pounds," or "I am eating healthy meals" or "I am fitting into my skinny jeans," etc.

9. **FINISH:** Write those statements on a fresh sheet of paper. These are your goals.

10. **SPEAK:** There's power in verbalizing things. Say your goals out loud.

#5 *Add Some Secret Sauce*

Now that you have vocalized your goals, your mind has clarity. You know what you want, so that brilliant brain of yours can focus and open your eyes to these forthcoming realities. But here's some real talk. At some point, your oomph is gonna fizzle out. I think we can agree that it's common to get all hot and heavy with something new like a steamy fling only to cast it aside when the initial spark is gone. It happens to all of us. That's where this secret sauce comes into play.

I want you to define your *Why*.

Think of it as your *Why Power*. It's your reason for being; your reason for doing what you're doing. Getting clear on your goals is one thing, but when you get clear on your *Why,* your purpose, then you have practically unstoppable power.

Your *Why* may be profound. Maybe you want to lose 170 pounds so that you can live to watch your children grow up. The deeper the *Why,* the more powerful it will be. But your *Why* doesn't have to be so dramatic, either. This is your life. Don't feel bad if your reason for wanting to get strong and toned isn't so you can kick down the door of a burning building and save a group of schoolchildren. If your *Why* is to look smoking hot on the beach during your vacation next month or to drop jaws at your wedding, then damn it, that's your *Why*. Embrace it. Own it. Use it to power through the tough times when your desire to sit on the couch and rewatch season 1 of *Orange Is the New Black* has beaten up your desire for flat abs.

It's going to happen. And that's okay. Discovering your *Why* can make all the difference between a goal realized and another failed "resolution."

The process for discovering your *Why* doesn't need to be complicated. Ready?

1. Grab a fresh sheet of paper and a pen and look over your goals.
2. Ask yourself *why* you're after them.
3. Start writing the thoughts that come to mind. Just scribble away to your heart's content. Spend some time with this and force yourself to prod a little deeper with each reason.
4. Review what you wrote.
5. Pick the *most compelling reasons,* the ones that make you want to leap out of your chair right now and crush one of your workouts.
6. Write those reasons down on a fresh piece of paper.
7. Make copies and put them everywhere you can see. The fridge, your desk, the bathroom mirror. You can even make it the background on your phone! Anywhere that you're going to look, put one so that you can remind yourself why you're doing this.

#6 *Chart a Course*

All right, you know *what* you want and have powerful reasons for *why* you want it. Now it's time to figure out *how* you're going to get there.

The trouble with goals, even if we make them super-specific, is that on their own they're nothing more than statements of desire. How do you actually go about *getting* them? This takes a strategy and action. Again, let's keep this simple.

1. **REVIEW:** Look at your goals.
2. **IDENTIFY:** Remember when I said that a habit is nothing more than a behavior that's become ingrained over time by the choices we make on a daily basis? We're now going to

identify *which* behaviors you need to incorporate day to day. These behaviors, when repeated over time, will become habits and those habits will lead you to achieve your goals. Ask yourself, "What do I need to do every day when I wake up to achieve my goals?"

Example

Goal: I am losing fat and gaining muscle tone.

- **Daily Behaviors:**
  - I am getting out of bed when my alarm first goes off.
  - I am drinking a glass of water with fresh-squeezed lemon upon waking.
  - I am thinking of three things I'm grateful for right now as I'm drinking my water and brushing my teeth.
  - I am doing my workout each morning before I leave the house.
  - I am enjoying a clean, lean breakfast after my workout.
  - I am eating five clean meals a day (breakfast, snack, lunch, snack, dinner).
  - If I want a treat, I am cutting out one snack and replacing it with an indulgence capped at around 200 calories.
  - I am getting up from my desk to stretch and/or take a short walk every hour. I am setting a calendar reminder to help me follow through on that.
  - I am taking all of my phone calls standing up.
  - I am "unplugging" two hours before bed without phones, Internet, or TV to unwind and prepare myself for bed.
  - I am getting 7–8 hours of quality sleep every night.

- **Weekly Behaviors:**
  - I am completing all five workouts, plus Recovery Yoga, and resting fully on Sundays.
  - I am planning my meals for the week on Sunday, assembling a grocery list, and going shopping to best prepare myself for a week of great eating.
  - I am seeking out one new fun and active thing to do this week and putting it on my calendar.
  - I am replacing half the time I spend watching TV each night with an activity that enriches my mind.
  - I am connecting with other people who are leading healthy, active lives at least once this week in order to build a strong and supportive community.

3. **WRITE IT DOWN:** Get these ideas out of your head and onto paper. Put them places that you'll see every day. That will remind you of what you're supposed to be doing and keep you motivated. Ideas swimming around in your head can all too easily become fantasies. Write them down and ensure that they become actions.

4. **DO IT. AGAIN AND AGAIN AND AGAIN:** A behavior becomes a habit only after it's been repeated long enough. Again, twenty-one days seems to be the habit-forming time period. At first, these steps and new behaviors may feel a bit robotic and mechanical, forced even. That's totally normal. This is a deliberate and thoughtful way of instilling a new, positive lifestyle. Just stick with it. It may take more effort to get and keep the ball rolling when you start, but I promise that if you maintain your daily and weekly behaviors, before long you'll catch a tailwind and those things that took so much

effort to start and sustain will simply become a normal part of your everyday life.

#7 *Love the Haters*

Have you ever tried to do something positive for yourself, but the people around you seem intent on blocking you at every turn? It happens. And it might happen during this six-week program. As frustrating as it may be, I have to remind you to look at Key #1. Stop blaming others.

This journey is about you. Haters gonna hate, so don't get angry if your family and friends aren't supportive at first, or maybe even at all. Keep your eyes set squarely on your goals and let your behaviors be driven by your *Why*.

Now let's get real. You're at a meeting where there are several trays of cookies. Your coworker Craig offers you one, which you politely decline. Maybe he shrugs and the tray keeps moving, but maybe he pries a little, asking if you're on a diet.

"No, not a diet," you say. "I'm doing this six-week fitness challenge, but basically I just try to eat healthy and stick to indulgences that I *really* enjoy."

The next thing you know, that plate of cookies has somehow made its way right back in front of you. You're thinking, *That asshole purposely put those cookies right in front of me, knowing damn well I'm trying not to eat them!*

As much as you'd like to reach across the table and knock him into next week, there's a better way. You can take a Zen approach and simply be still, acknowledging what's happening and refusing to engage in a destructive way. Or you can also channel this frustration you're feeling and let it drive you to push harder toward your goals. You can even go for a combo of the two. Craig the Cookie Pusher? Ignore him. He has his own issues. Put your focus on yourself and ignore the little punk.

Let the haters hate. Stay strong and focused. You have far bigger fish to grill.

#8 *Get Some Backup*

A strong community is a great way to keep yourself accountable and motivated. Recruit your friends and family on your journey. It's only six weeks, but I have a feeling that by the time you finish this program, you'll look at this less as a "challenge" and more as a lifestyle that you can embrace forever.

But if your friends and family aren't into joining, what's a person to do? Sure, you could do a "friend cleanse" and kick your crew to the curb as you go off in search of an enlightened group of fitness fanatics, but that's advice that sounds good on paper but is, obviously, impractical.

The one caveat here is to be mindful of truly poisonous relationships. It's one thing for someone to be reluctant to join in on a six-week fitness program, but it's another for them to sabotage you and tear you down. If there are people like this in your life, it's time to bounce. Their presence isn't doing you an ounce of good. Maybe one day you can revisit the relationship, but right now it's got to go.

If you absolutely can't get this person or these people out of your life, my advice is to start slow, be honest, and have a few difficult conversations. Tell them what your goals are, that you're on this six-week program not just to get in shape, but to live a truly healthy, inspired life. This isn't a diet fad, but a lifestyle you're embracing, and you need their support. Be as specific as you can. Spell out for them exactly what you need. If they won't play ball, then tell them you can't be around them. Sometimes people need a cold dose of reality. This may be a physically and emotionally uncomfortable conversation, but more times than not, it works.

At the same time, start to seek out people who share some of your newfound interests. Is there someone at work who you've noticed eats really well? Strike up a conversation. Tell them that you've noticed they always seem to be eating super-clean at the office and you're on this six-week program and blah, blah, blah. You may have just made a friend who can help keep you accountable on your journey.

And don't forget, even if your friends and family won't take this six-week journey with you, there are a ton of people around the country who are doing this program right now. Why not connect with some of them? Search the hashtag 30SB on social media. Reach out and make some friends. I can tell you firsthand that the bonds of friendship forged in sweat last a long time!

#9 Be Happy Now

Far too many of us live with a set of "when I" beliefs. I'll be happy *when I* lose twenty pounds. I'll be happy *when I* am making six figures.

The major difference between a set of "when I" beliefs and goals lies in self-acceptance, in being happy with what you have and who you are now as you work toward creating the life you want. It's realizing that you're no less whole before achieving a goal than after you've achieved it.

It's critical to know that you are perfect *right now*. Any work you do to achieve a goal of any kind is simply enhancing that.

It may seem like a subtle difference, semantics even, but it's a radical shift in mentality that can positively impact the way you view yourself and approach life. And I promise it makes the attainment of your goals even sweeter.

As any study or book on positive psychology will tell you, the big trouble with this "when I" recipe for happiness that most of us have is that it just creates a perpetual cycle of *un*happiness. You chase after something and when you finally get it, what happens? You have a momentary surge of pleasure that quickly fades and is replaced by the desire for something new.

When I lose twenty pounds, I'll be happy, but when you lose those twenty pounds, your brain changes the definition of what happiness is.

I lost twenty pounds! Now I need to get a better job.

I got a better job. Now I need a promotion.

I got a promotion. Now I need to stop working so much and follow my true passion.

See the pattern here?

You've equated the definition of happiness with something outside yourself. Think about those old *Three Stooges* episodes where one of the characters would bend down to pick something up, only to kick it farther forward, just out of reach. It would go on and on till one of the other Stooges slapped him across the face and said, "Wake up, stupid!" This is kind of like that.

I know a lot of thin, toned people who are miserable, and plenty of overweight people who are radically happy. I also know a lot of extremely wealthy people who hate life and people with practically no money who live like kings. The difference isn't the number on the scale or the zeroes on the bank statement: It's the *mindset*.

So how do we get happy *now*? We cultivate happiness through gratitude and awareness in the present moment.

I'm not trying to get all New Agey on you here. This is something I've come to learn through personal experience over the years, often resisting the idea because I thought it was kind of silly. I now know better. Like they say, the proof is in the pudding.

As I said before: You are perfect right now, exactly as you are. If you find that difficult to believe, then you need to spend more time cranking up the self-love and dialing down the self-loathing. Speak kindly to yourself, be proud of your accomplishments, and never talk trash about your body.

As with everything else, you're not going to wave a magic wand and have an overnight transformation. This takes practice. You have to *choose* to *make it* a daily practice. To be proud of and grateful for who you are and all that your body is capable of today. Through daily practice it will become a habit, and when it becomes a habit, a funny thing happens: The engine kicks on and you redline it straight through the finish line and keep going.

Some strategies I've learned that can help you to be happy now:

- **MEDITATE DAILY:** this can be for as little as 5 minutes. Sit in silence somewhere you'll be free from distractions for the duration of your meditation, set a timer, then close your eyes and focus your attention on the tip of your nose, right outside your nostrils.

  Sit in a chair or on the floor. If you're on the floor, sit on a cushion or folded blanket so your hips are raised up. From here, observe your breath as it goes out and comes in. If your mind wanders or you get caught up in a thought, and this will happen, don't wrestle your mind back or try to drive the thoughts away. Just keep breathing and gently direct your attention back to the tip of your nose, where you'll simply observe the breath. When the timer goes off, take a nice deep breath and thank yourself for taking the time to quiet your mind and improve your life.

Developing the ability to sit in silence like this allows you to create deep states of concentration and contemplation and create stillness in your life. It also helps counteract the horrible habit we've developed of multitasking our brains into a forced state of ADD. Whether it's doing five things at once at the office or being unable to walk down the street without checking your Instagram, this practice is not serving your overall wellness. Meditation can help.

- **PRACTICE YOGA:** You're going to be doing yoga once a week as a way to enhance your mobility and keep your body limber, but a regular yoga practice has far greater benefits than physical elasticity. Yoga poses can be pretty uncomfortable. Practicing yoga forces us to be still and relaxed in moments of discomfort. That's a skill you can take off the mat and into your life.

- **GO OUTSIDE AND PLAY:** It's easy to lose perspective. Take a walk on the beach or in the woods and look around. Gazing out at the ocean or up at the stars or at an oak tree that's been enduring the changing seasons for more than a hundred years can help put some of our fairly petty problems and irritations in context. If you're in a city, think about the places you loved when you first moved there—neighborhoods, parks, dog runs, coffee shops—and go take a stroll.

- **FIND BALANCE:** I spoke about this with the Life360 Chart. Are you placing a heavy emphasis on one area of your life and neglecting others? If so, it will throw your life balance out of whack and create that nagging sense of daily irritation and unhappiness. Look at the chart and rate your happiness in each area on a scale of 1–10. Your numbers in each category should be roughly the same high level of happiness. If you notice one area that's particularly low, set goals in that area to help raise your happiness and then establish daily behaviors that will get you there.

- **GIVE GENEROUSLY:** No matter who you are, where you've come from, or how much money you make, everyone has *something* to give. Be it your time, resources, or both, put more emphasis on taking good care of others in ways that really matter. This one practice alone can change your life forever. And though it can't be proven in a lab, I can tell you from personal experience that you get out of this life what you give. For better or worse. Let's commit to ensuring it's for the better and find ways to start giving today.

#10 *Audit Yourself*

This program is six weeks, but like I've been saying, this isn't a fad diet or crash plan. It's a blueprint for a happy, healthy lifestyle. With that in mind, I'd like you to perform a quarterly checkup. Every three months, take a few hours to sit and review your state of affairs.

Ask yourself:

- Am I where I want to be physically?
- Do I feel strong, energetic, and vibrant?
- Am I keeping up with my daily behaviors?
- Do my goals need to be adjusted in any way?
- Am I happy?

Revisit that Life360 Chart whenever you need to. Setting goals and tailoring your behaviors to get where you want to go should be a fun, lifelong process. It may not always be easy, but it should be simple.

And always remember, the winners in this fitness game aren't the ones who lose weight the fastest. They're the ones who keep it off the longest. You, friend, are going to keep it off for life.

And that life starts right now. You've taken the time to read this book, to do the workouts, and to follow the keys. I can't possibly begin to tell you how proud I am of you for all the hard work you've done so far and all the great things you've yet to do.

This isn't the end of the road. Far from it. You've started down a path that is going to take you places you may have only dreamed about, and that hot body of yours is the vehicle.

And we're not parting ways just yet. This may be the last page of this book, but I'm still right here with you. Right now. Let's connect! Drop me an email. Reach out to me on social media. Come by one of my events sometime and say hi. If you'll have me, I'd be truly honored to be a consistent part of your life. Now let's set the book down, get out there, and live hard!

ACKNOWLEDGMENTS

MARNIE COCHRAN. YOU ARE A MAGIC-MAKER and an author's dream come true. Thank you for making this journey so much fun and for bringing out the best in me!

Dave Zinczenko and Stephen Perrine. Thank you and Zinc Ink for helping make this journey possible.

Nina Shield. Thank you for your expert eye and guidance.

Joy Tutela. You are *far* more than a literary agent; you are a true collaborator and consigliera.

David Black. Your sage advice is absolutely priceless.

The entire team at Random House and Zinc Ink at every level. It takes a village. Our village is pretty awesome.

Alanna Kaivalya from alannak.com for helping to bring the yoga section of this book to life. You help keep me mobile, flexible, and humble. Xo.

Lisa Held, Melisse Gelula, and Alexia Brue from wellandgoodnyc .com. I'll never be able to thank you enough for all you've done for me and all you do for so many. And Lisa, once again, because you're so amazing. Love you.

Marissa Stephenson and Jaclyn Emerick. I heart you both forever and a day.

Liz Plosser. You're a champion, a genius, and, most important, a friend.

Meredith Engel. My very first piece of press came from your thoughtful pen, er, keyboard. Yes, I know you were just doing your job, but an infinite round of thanks to you.

The city of New Orleans for inspiring me to start The People's Bootcamp and the city of New York for giving it a home.

About the Author

ADAM ROSANTE serves simple, yet ridiculously effective, fitness, nutrition, and life advice with a sense of humor. He's known for his unique ability to make complicated and overwhelming information remarkably less so.

That's why real people turn to him again and again to get in shape and live healthy, active, inspired lives.

Named one of the sexiest trainers in the country by *Self* magazine and one of the six hottest trainers to watch by *Details,* Adam has become a fixture in magazines, on TV shows, and in blogs, but is as easygoing and accessible as one of your crazy best friends.

Though you can see him and his tips in some of the glossiest magazines in print and on top-rated shows on television, he's proudest that when you google him, you'll find things like this from people across the country:

"This dude seems awesome . . . and so genuine . . . and offers real, authentic advice that is dogma-free."—Shira Engel, college student. Quote posted on her blog after she discovered Adam's nutrition advice in a *Well+Good* feature story.

In 2012, he founded The People's Bootcamp, a pay-what-you-can fitness brand that is often referred to as the hardest workout in New York and that *Elle* magazine calls "a populist antidote to the tyranny of $35 spin sessions." It led *Well+Good* to dub him "the city's very own fitness Che."

Adam is also the creator of WaveShape, a surf-inspired, equipment-free workout that he designed for surfer friends and then made available to all for free online. It's used every day by thousands of people around the world from Montana to Morocco. Check it out at www.getinwaveshape.com.

In 2013 he went on the *Today* show for the first time and taught Kathie Lee and Hoda a radically effective workout using . . . wine. It showed more than two million viewers that you don't have to take yourself so seriously or live a boring, restrictive life for it to be a healthy one.

Because he knows that people would rather spend time laughing with friends and family than suffer in a gym, his tips and advice cut through the clutter and help people get in amazing shape, in body and mind, *fast*.

As a result of Adam's popularity and sensible, accessible approach to fitness, wellness, and life, Target enlisted him as the brand ambassador for its wildly popular C9 apparel line.

Adam was born on Long Island and lives in Manhattan and Montauk with his wife, Kate, and their kitten, Annie, who was rescued from a boatyard.

He is certified as a fitness trainer and nutrition coach through the International Sports Sciences Association and holds a Level 1 Crossfit Trainer Certification. Most important, he knows that you are stronger than you think and capable of absolutely anything.

30-SECOND BODY 6-Week Workout Calendar

	Monday	Tuesday	Wednesday	Thursday	Friday	Saturday	Sunday
Week 1	Photos and Measurements 1 Fit Test 1	Cardio Blaze	Airborne	Recovery Yoga	Fire Power	Airborne	Pure Rest
Week 2	Cardio Blaze	Fire Power	Airborne	Recovery Yoga	Cardio Blaze	Fire Power	Pure Rest
Week 3	Fit Test 2	Airborne	Fire Power	Recovery Yoga	Cardio Blaze	Airborne	Photos and Measurements 2 —— Pure Rest
Week 4	Cardio Blaze	Airborne	Fire Power	Recovery Yoga	Fire Power	Cardio Blaze	Pure Rest
Week 5	Airborne	Cardio Blaze	Fire Power	Recovery Yoga	Cardio Blaze	Airborne	Pure Rest
Week 6	Fire Power	Airborne	Cardio Blaze	Recovery Yoga	Airborne	Fit Test 3	Photos and Measurements 3 —— Pure Rest

* Available as a printout at www.the30secondbody.com.